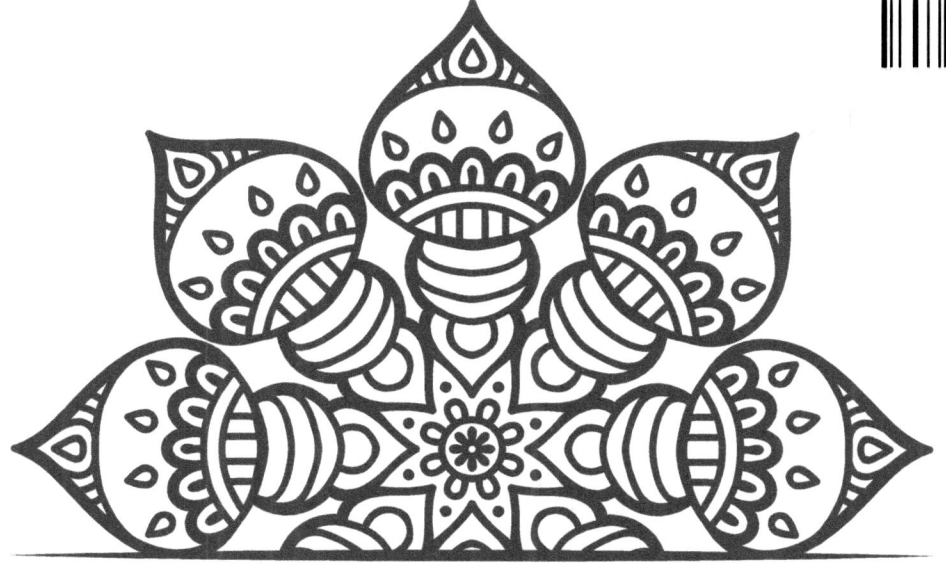

This Book Belongs To:

_____

_____

COLOR TEST
TEST YOUR COLOR SUPPLIES ON THIS PAGE TO SEE HOW THEY REACT TO THE PAPER.
PLACE A BLANK PAGE OR TWO BEHIND EACH PAGE AS YOU COLOR,
TO PREVENT BLEEO-THROUGH TO THE NEXT PAGE.

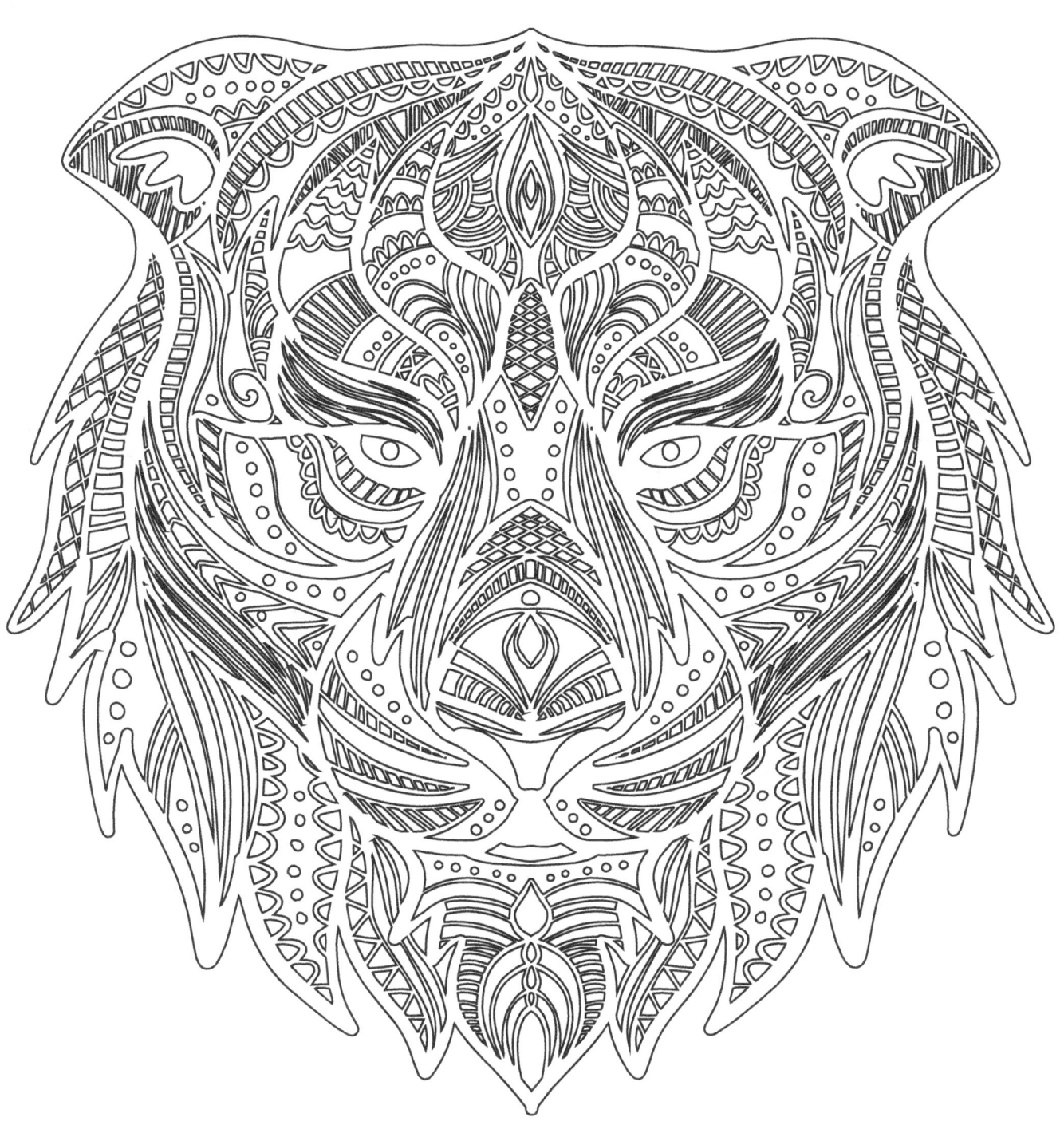

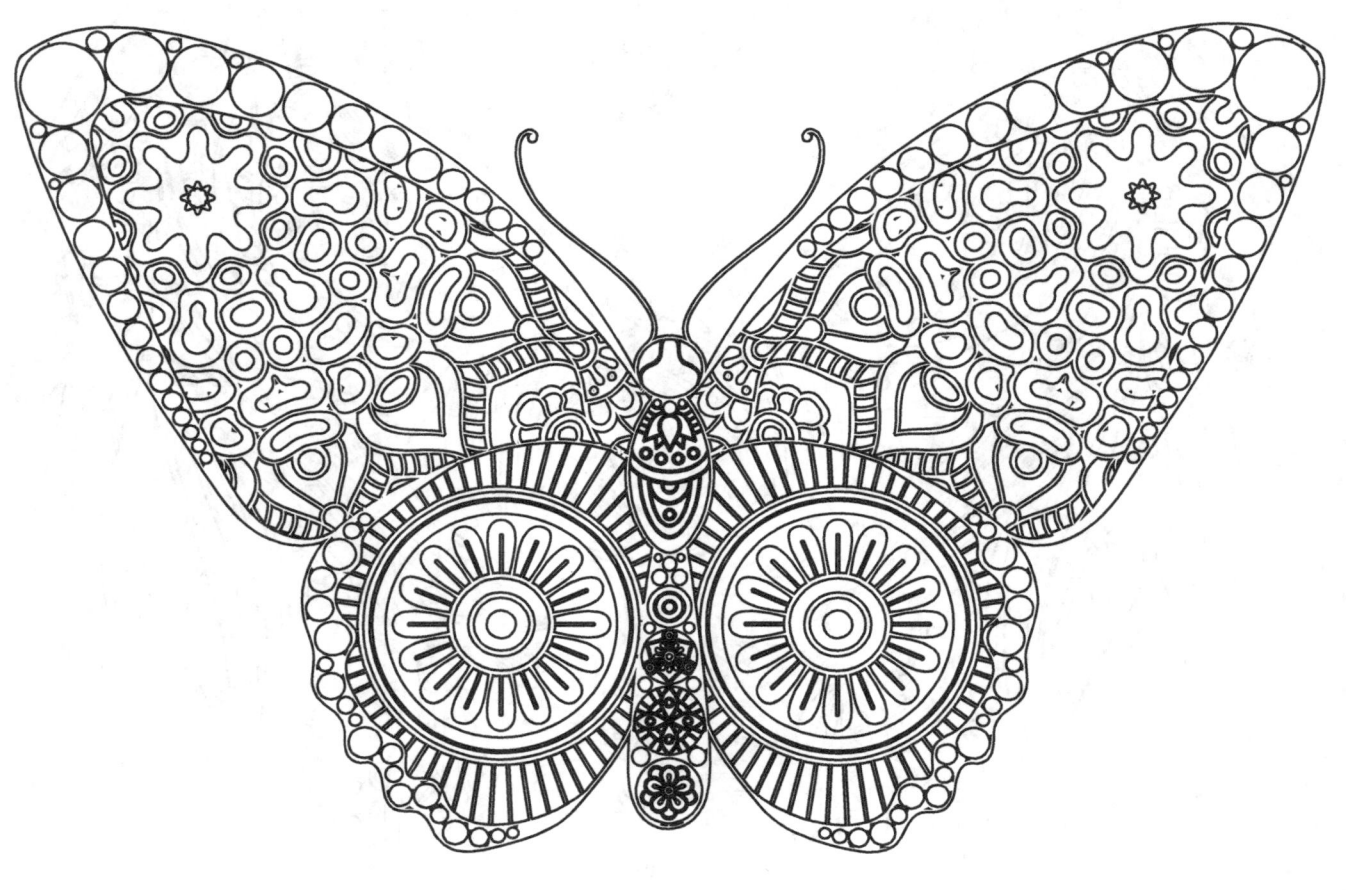

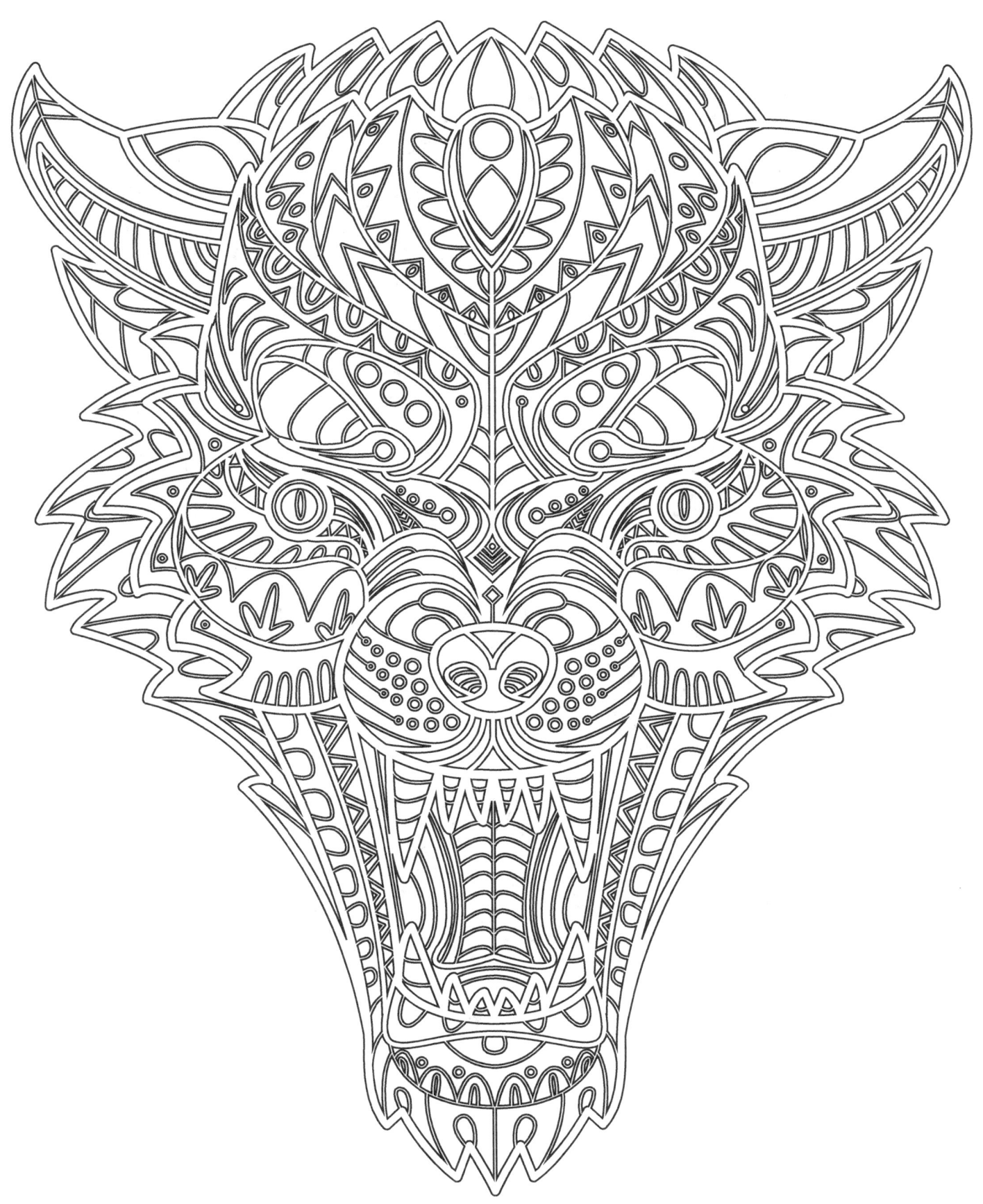

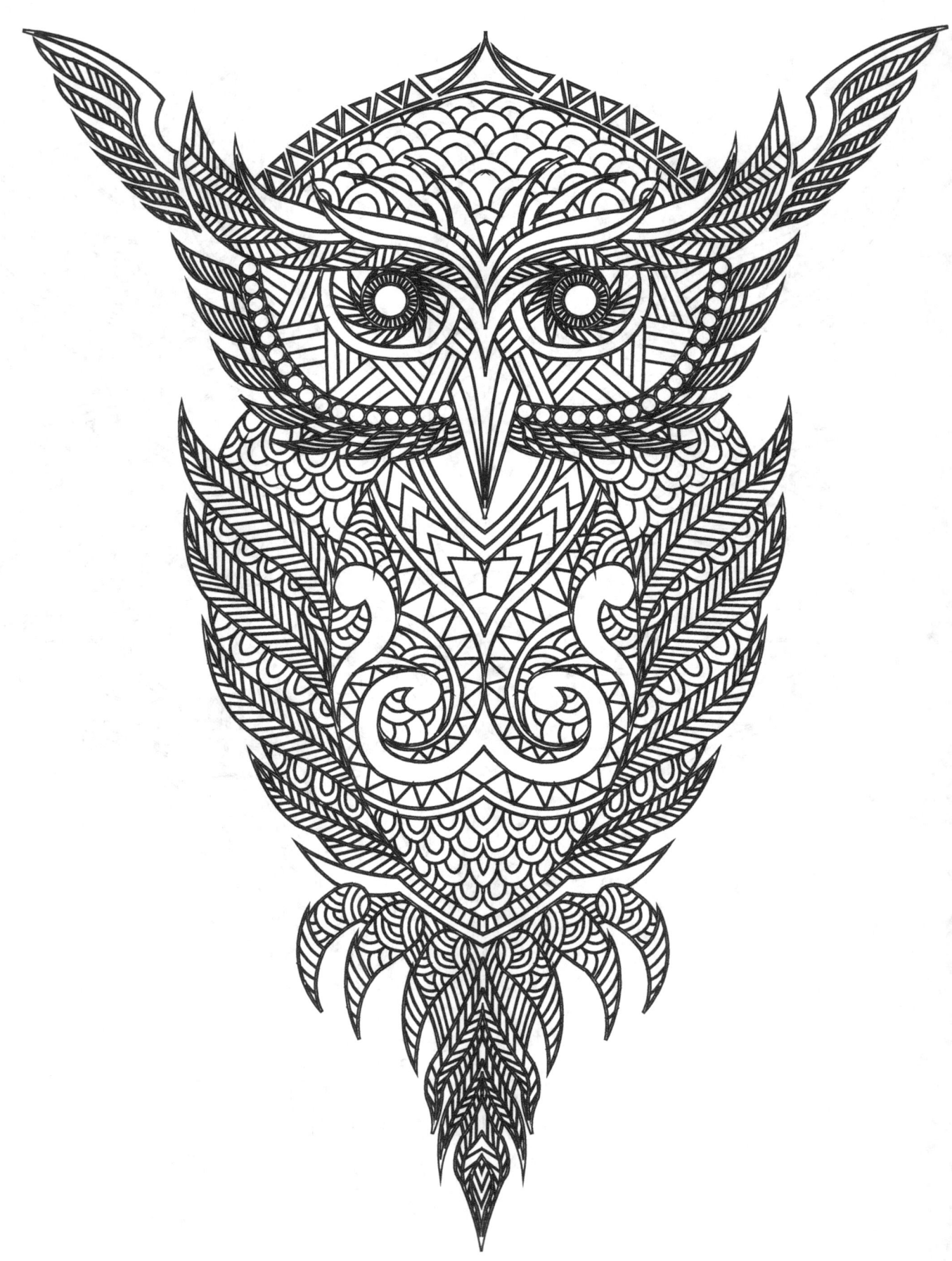

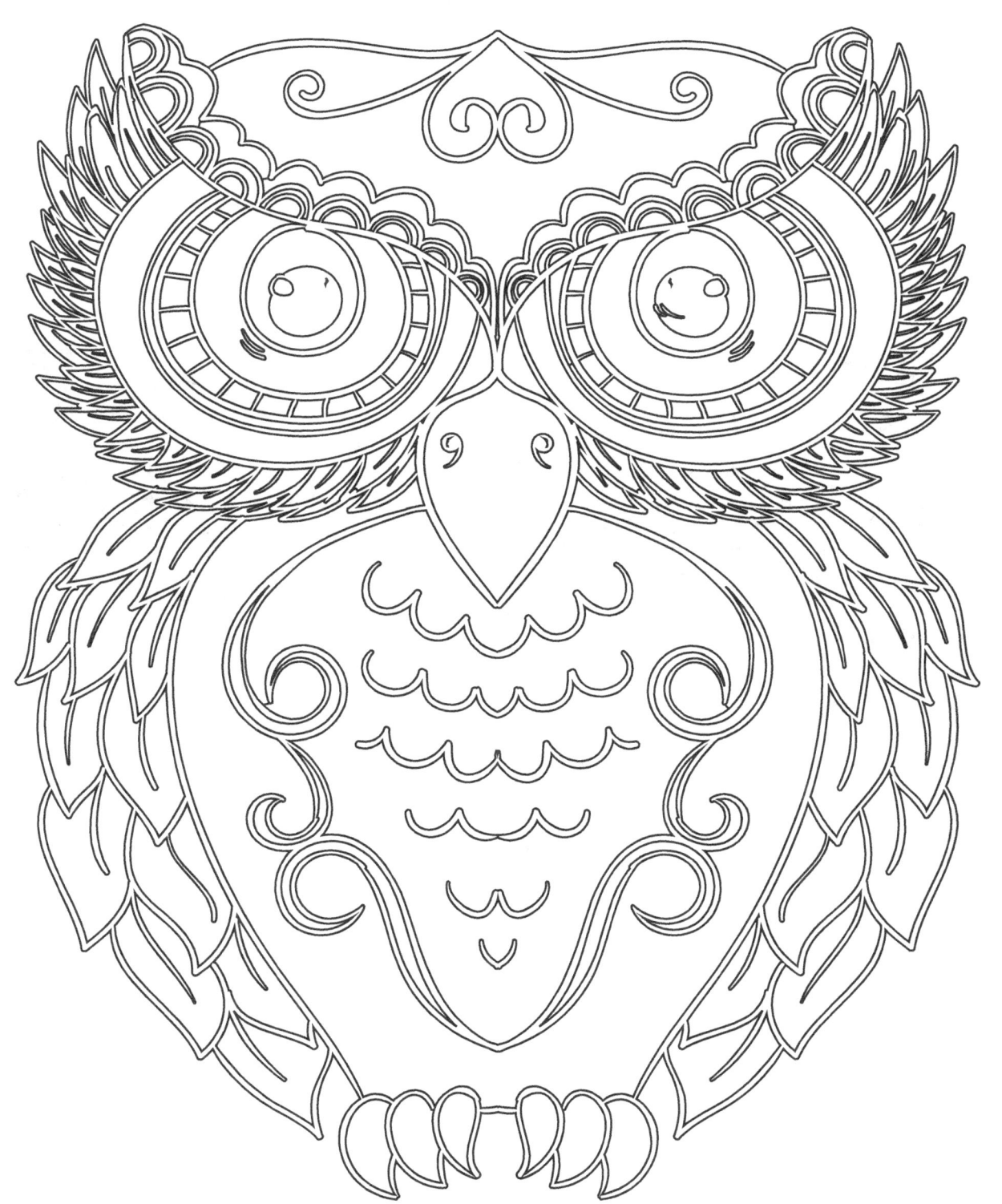

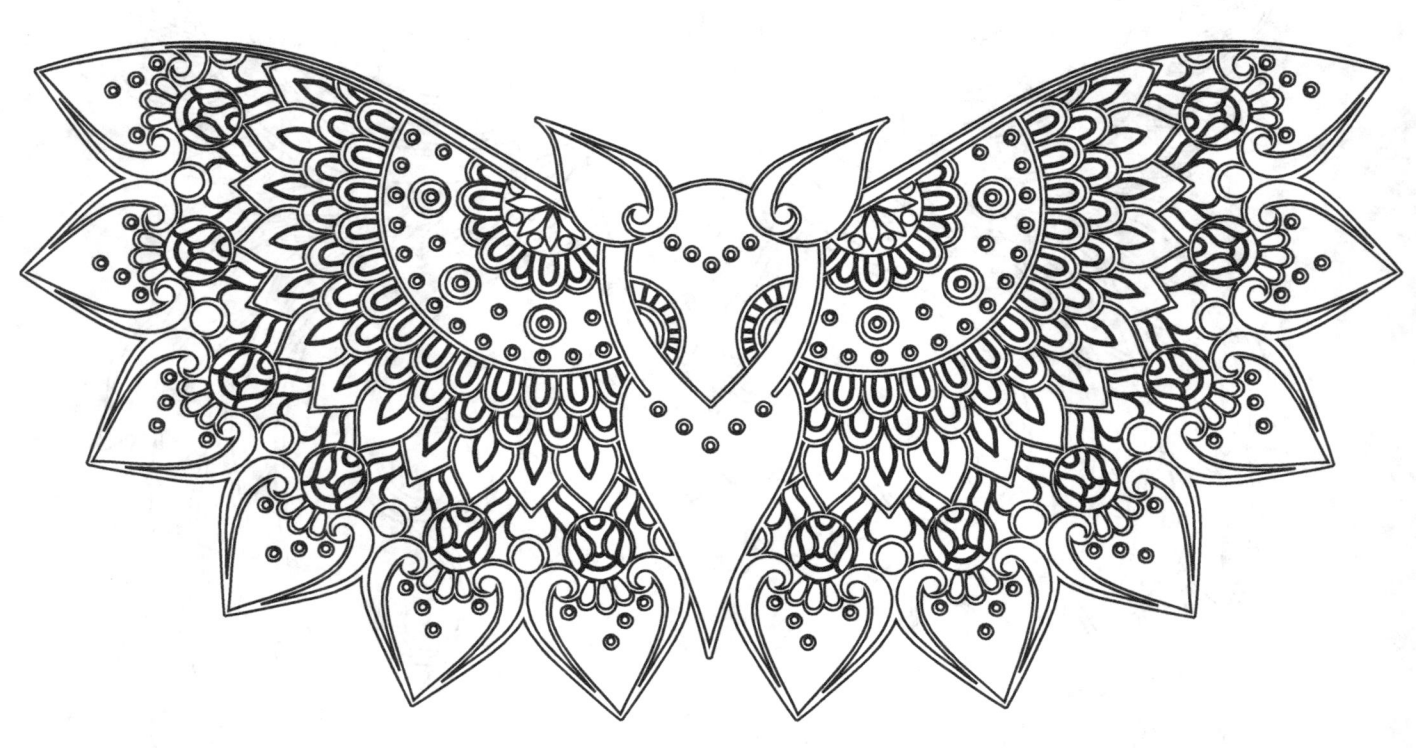

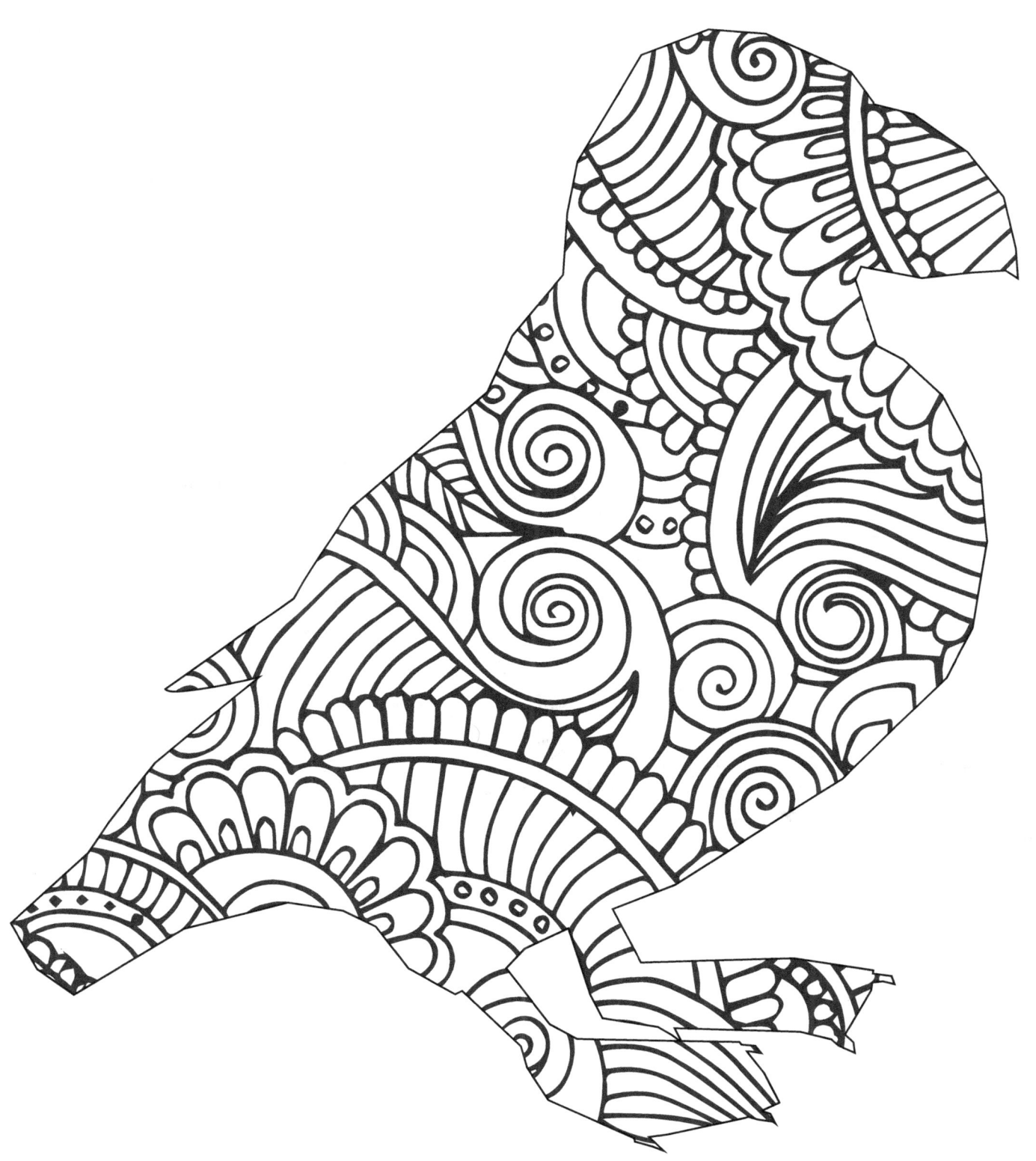

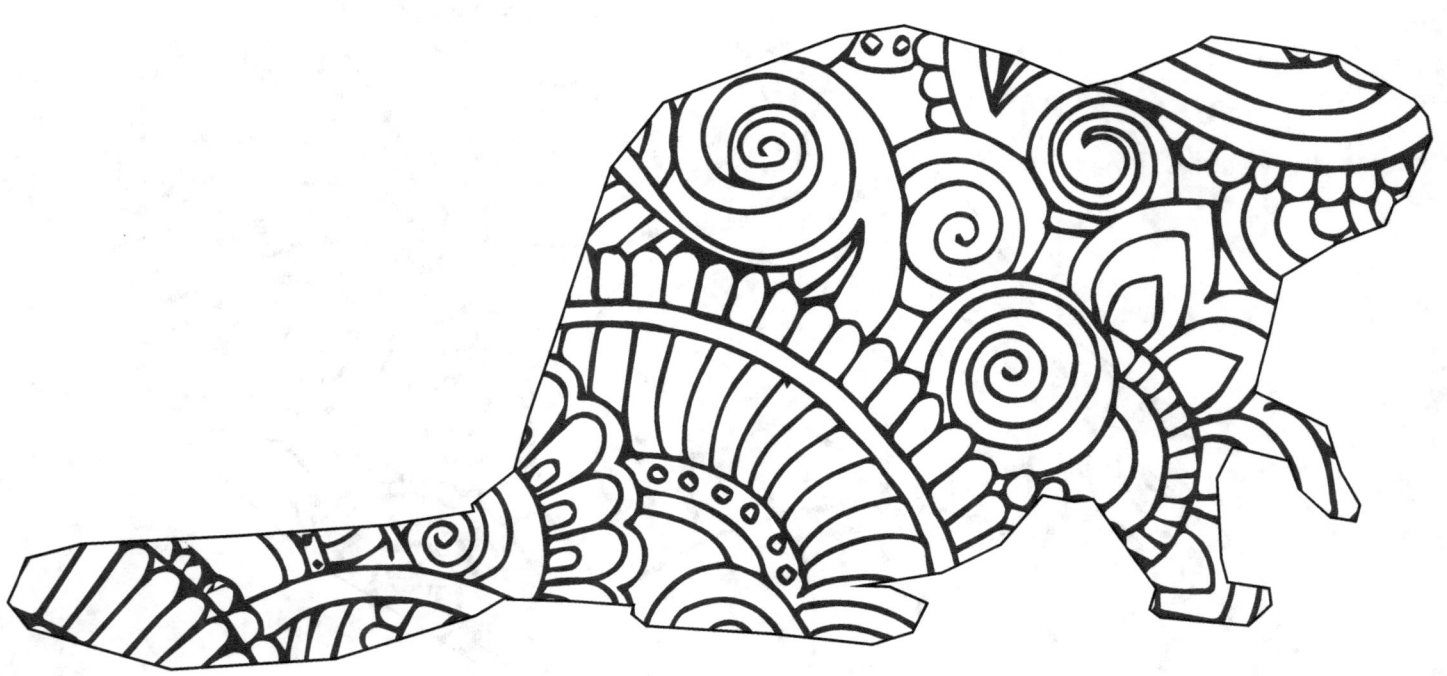

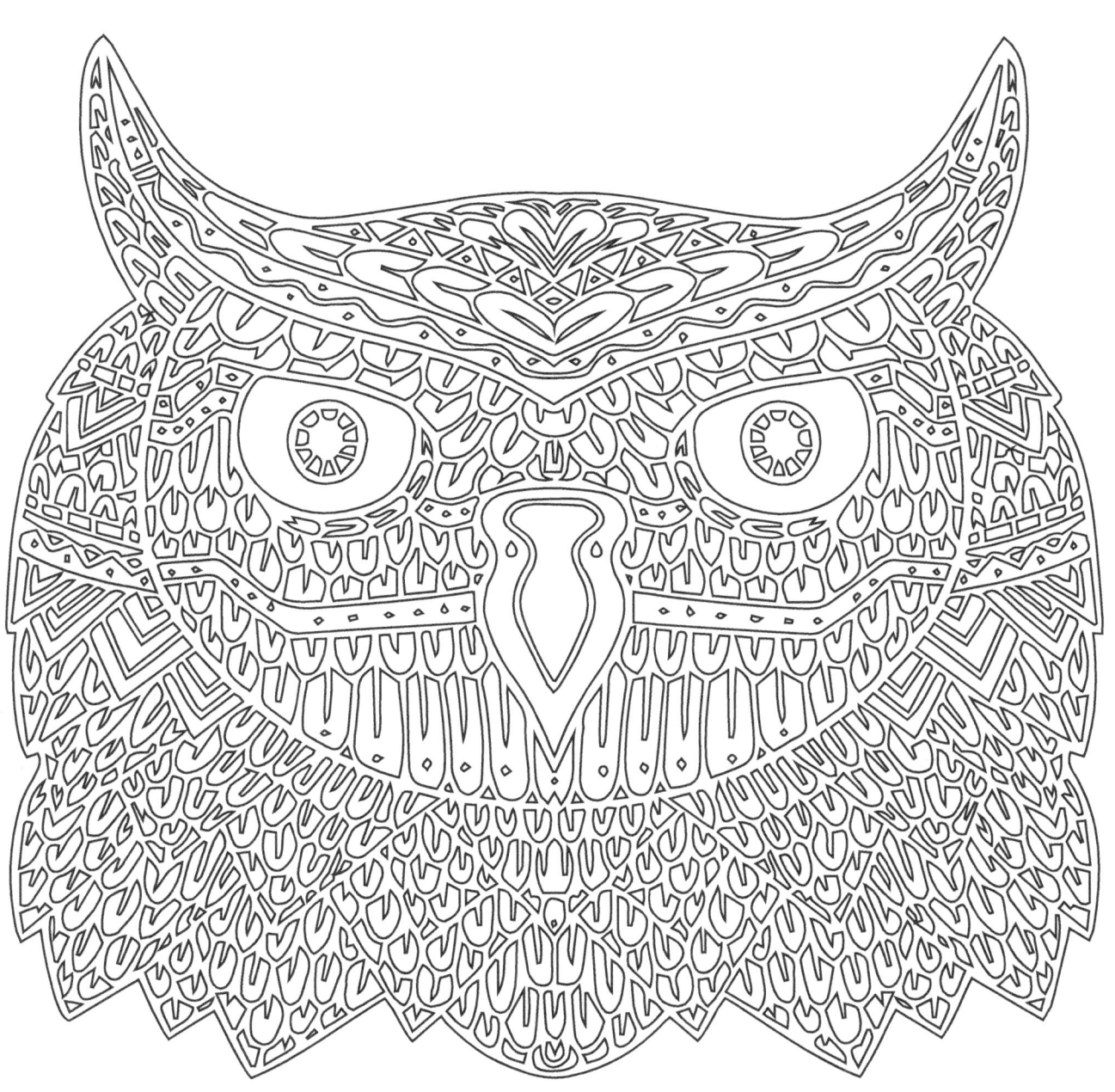

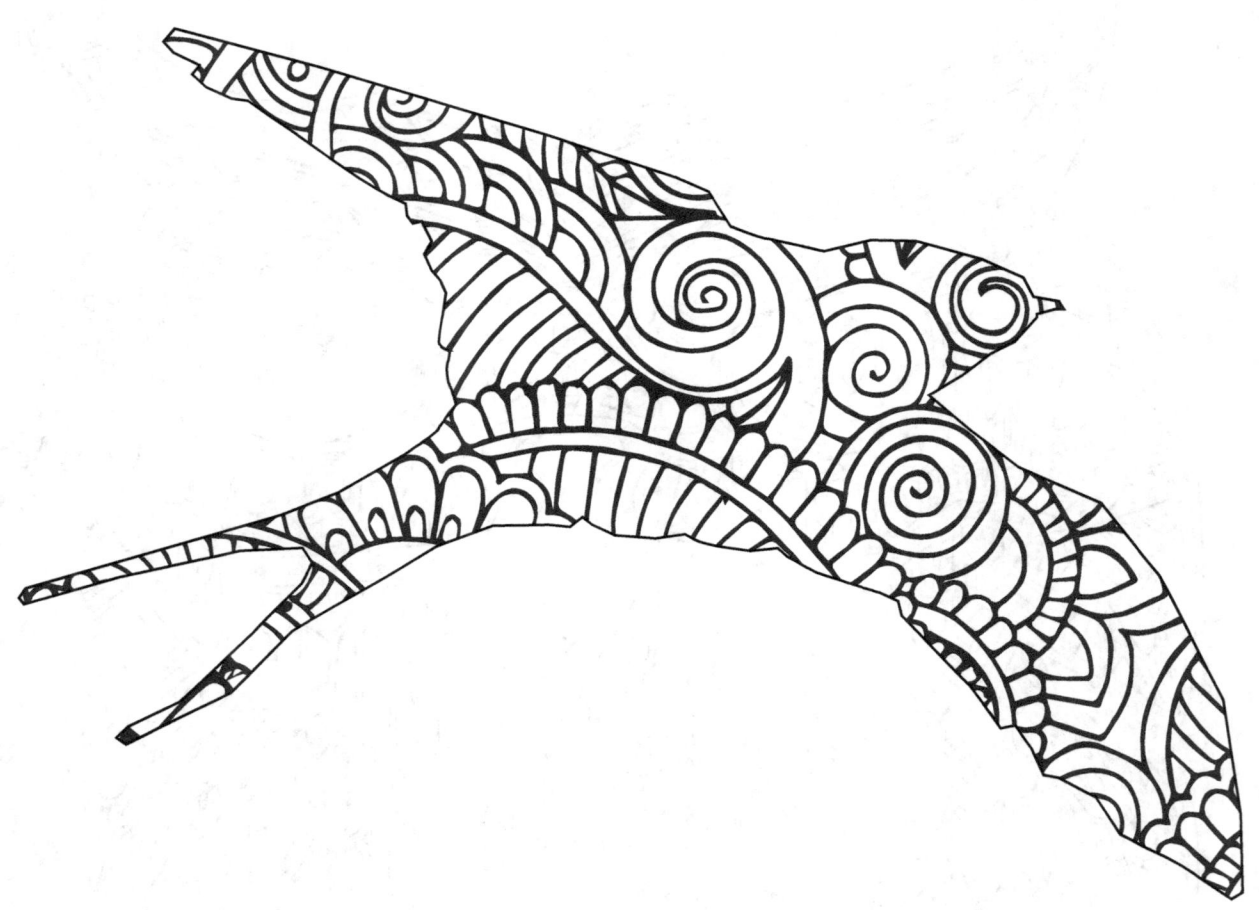

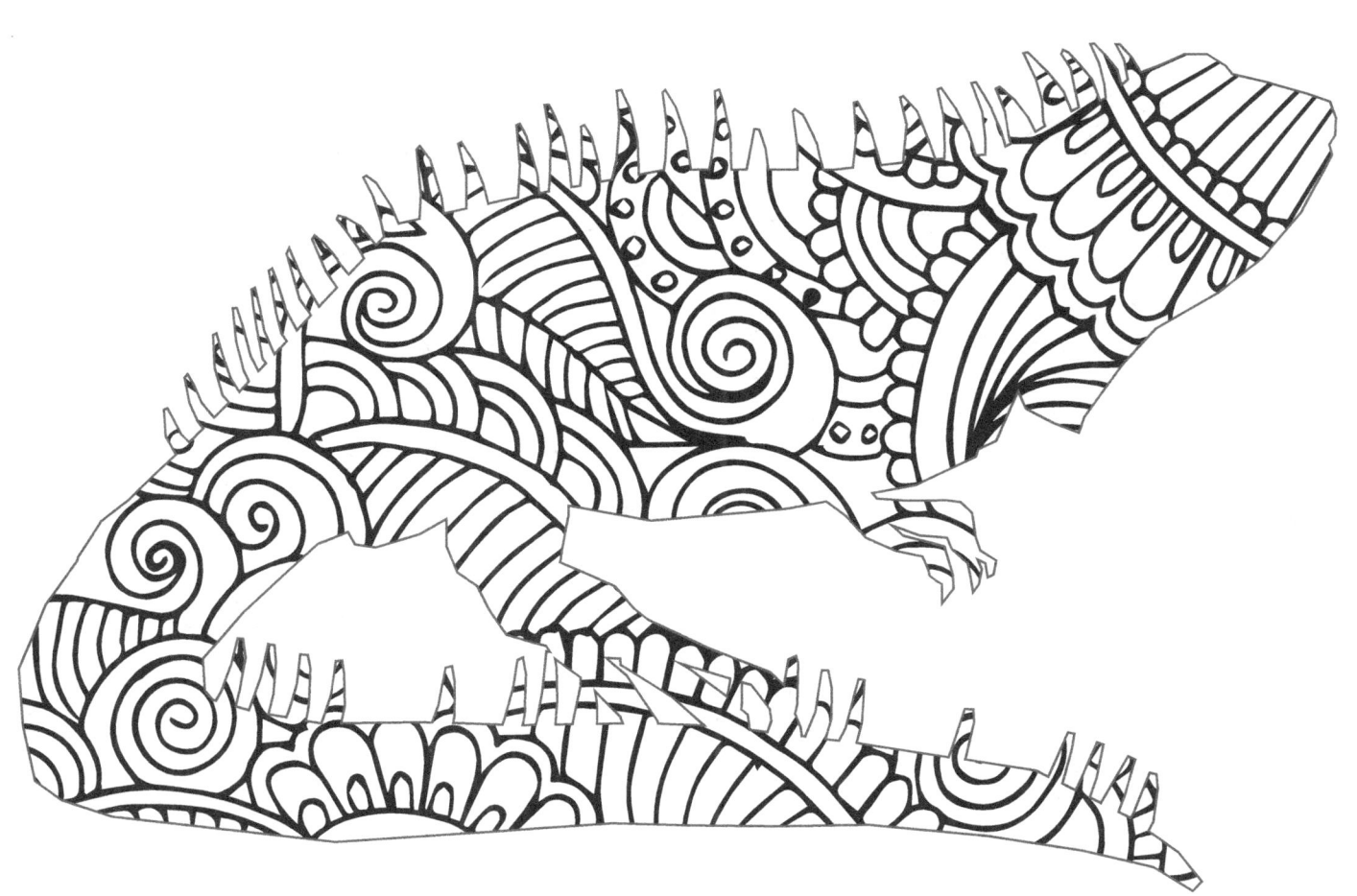

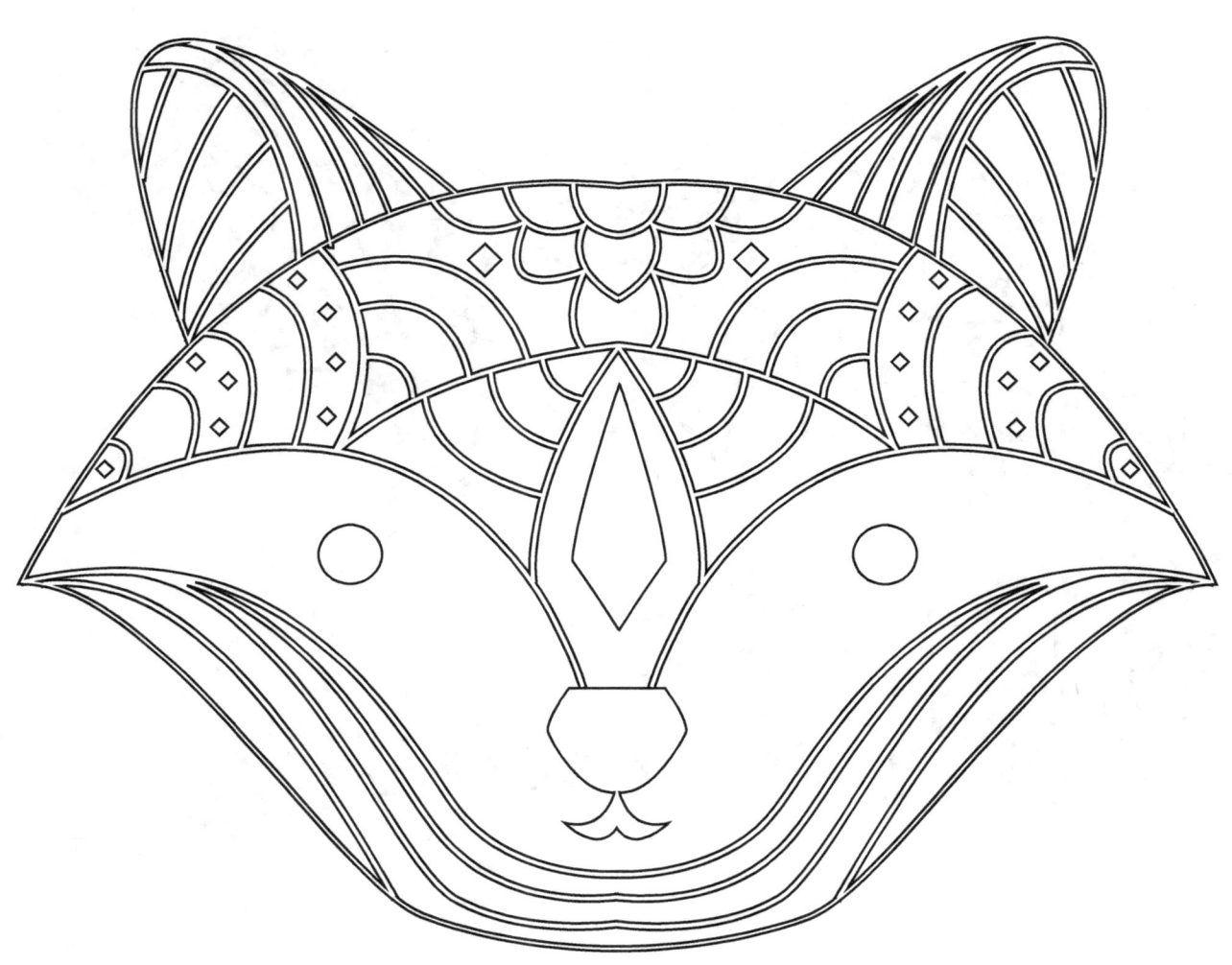

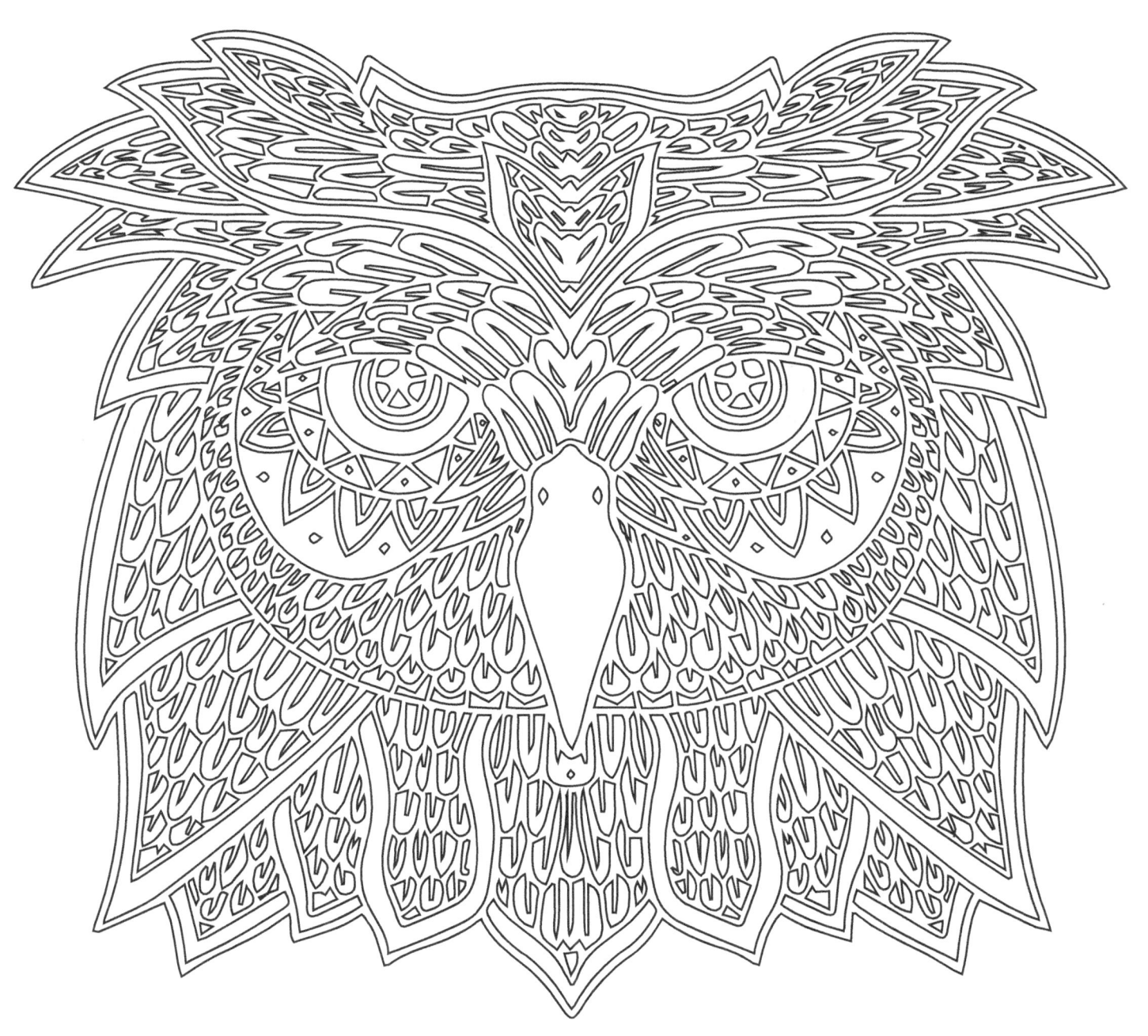

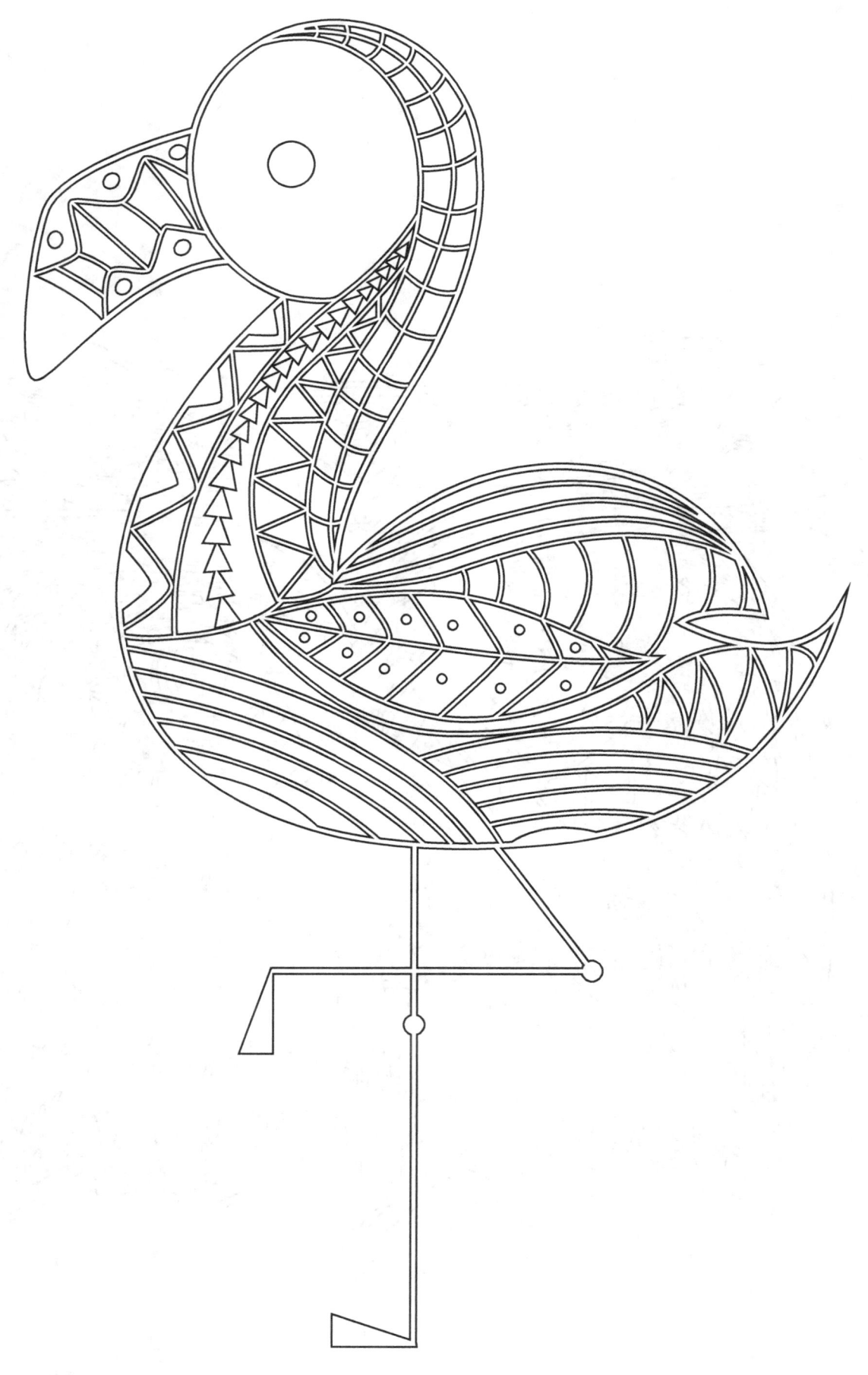

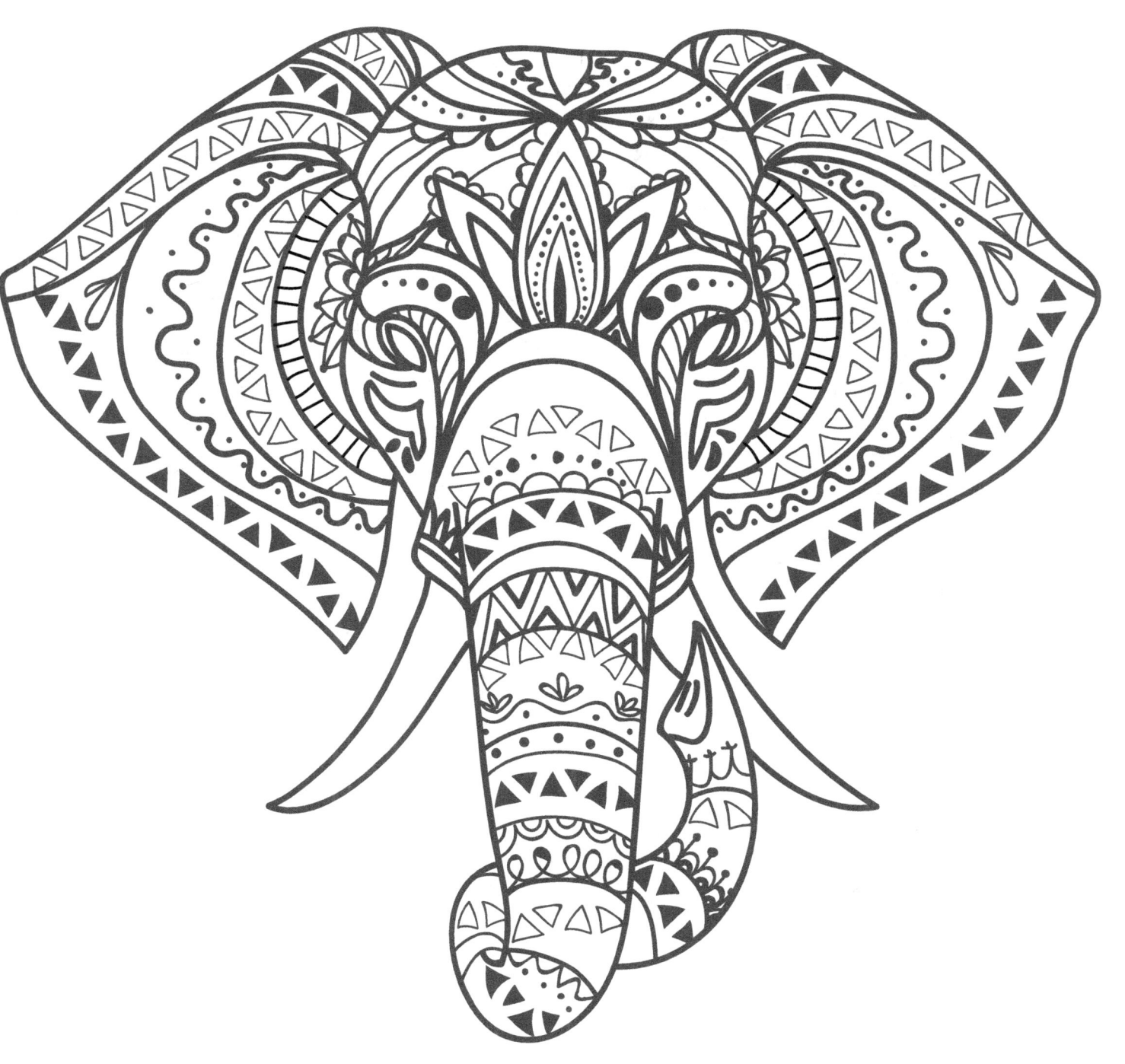

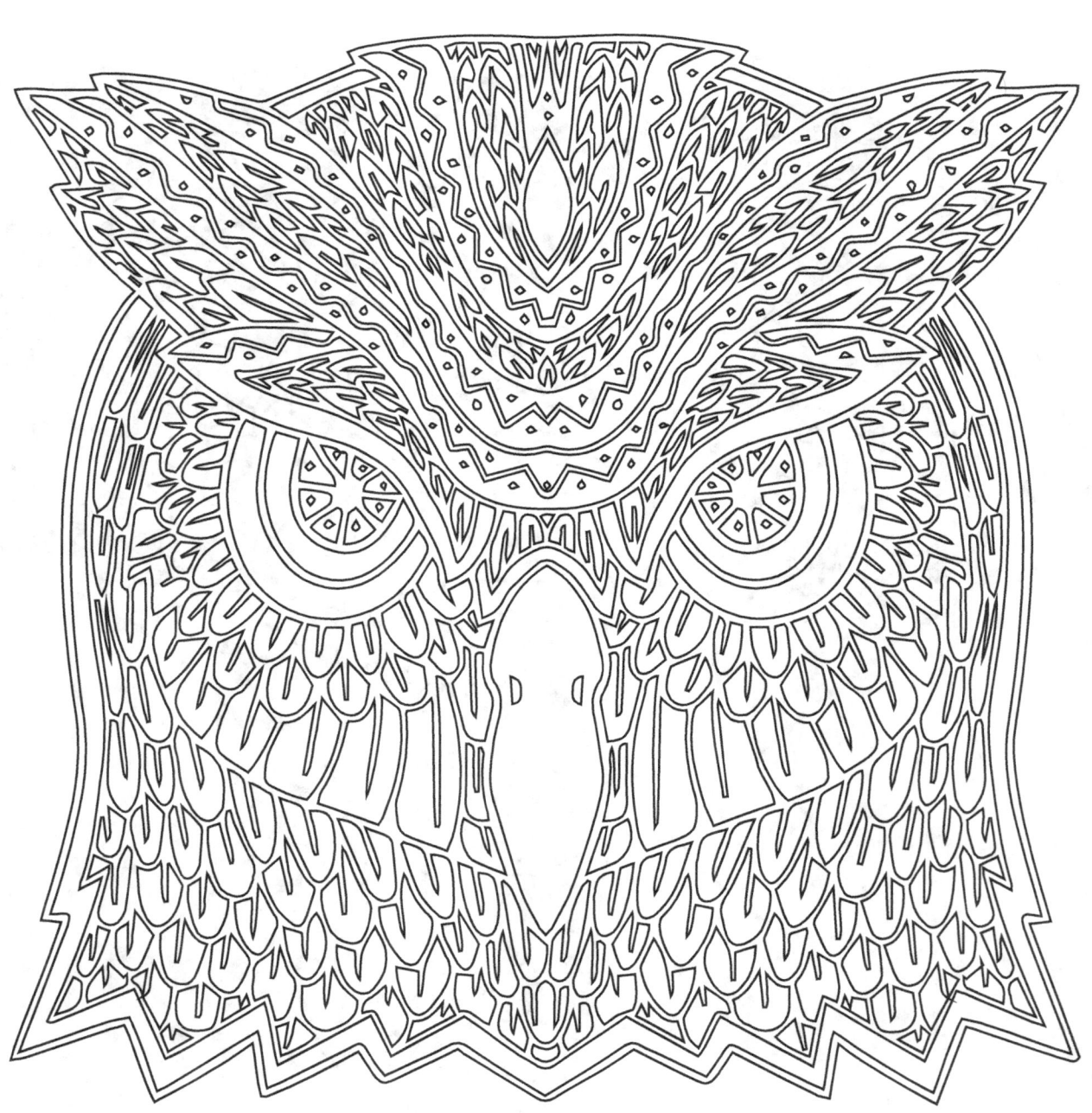

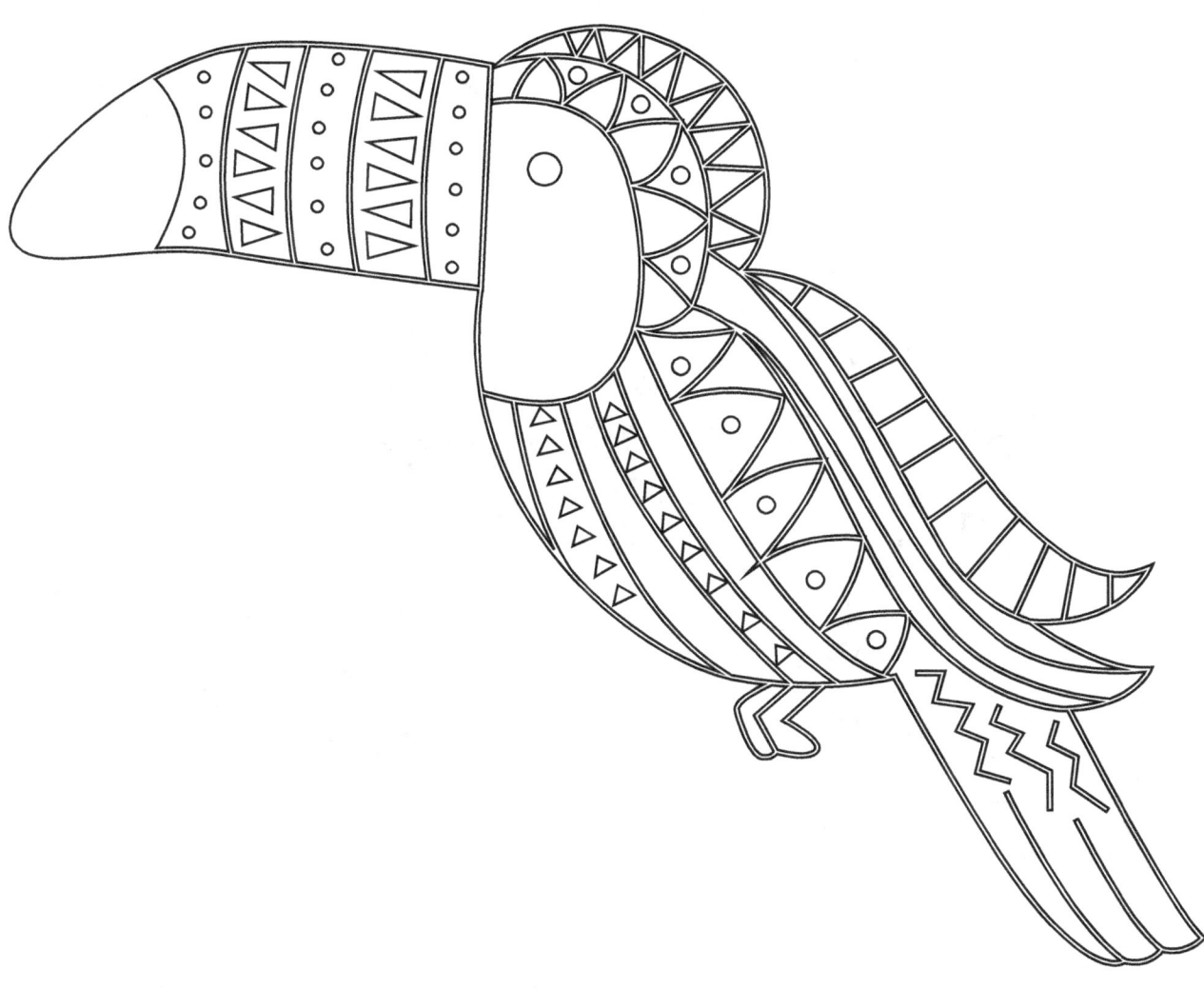

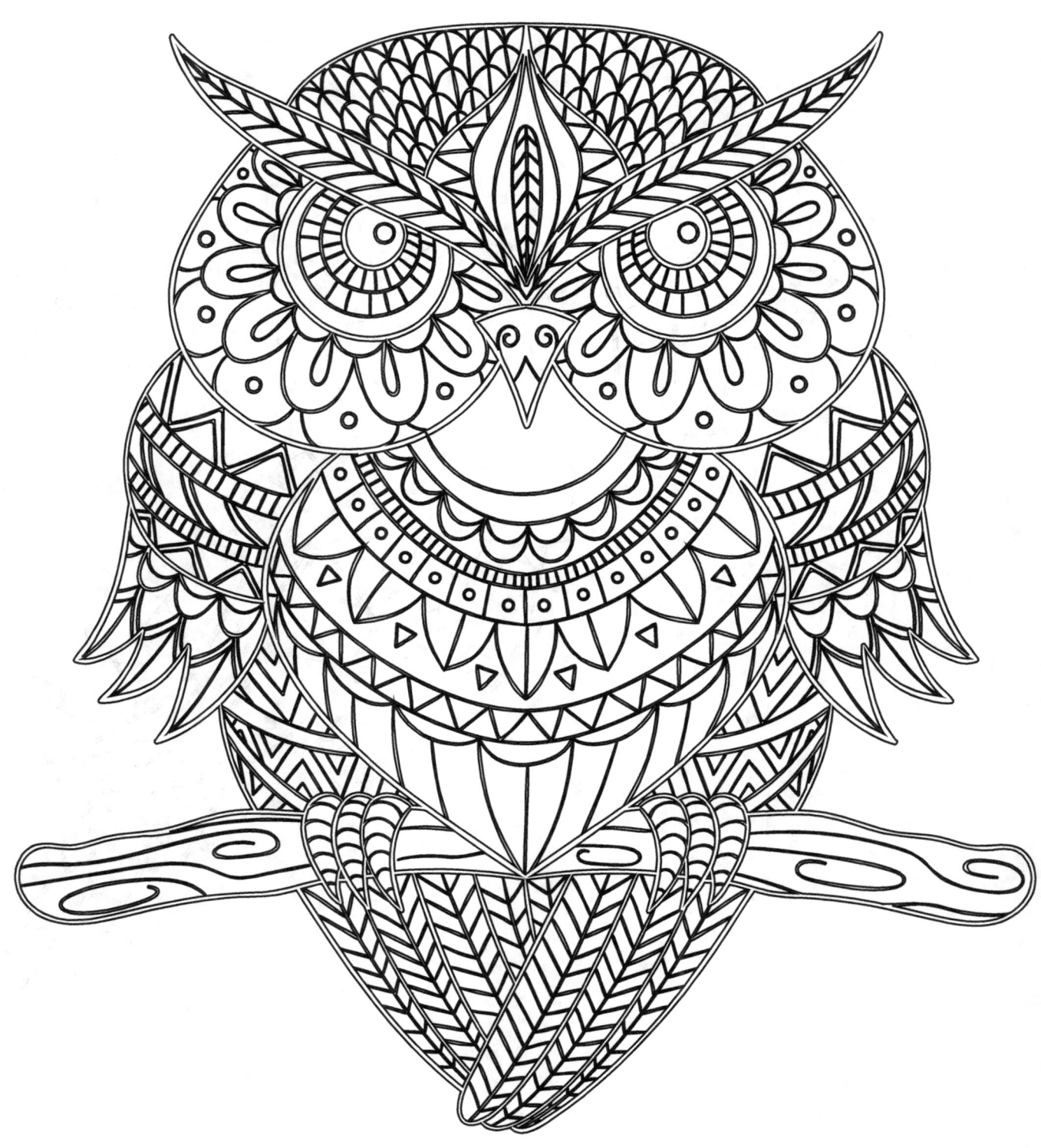

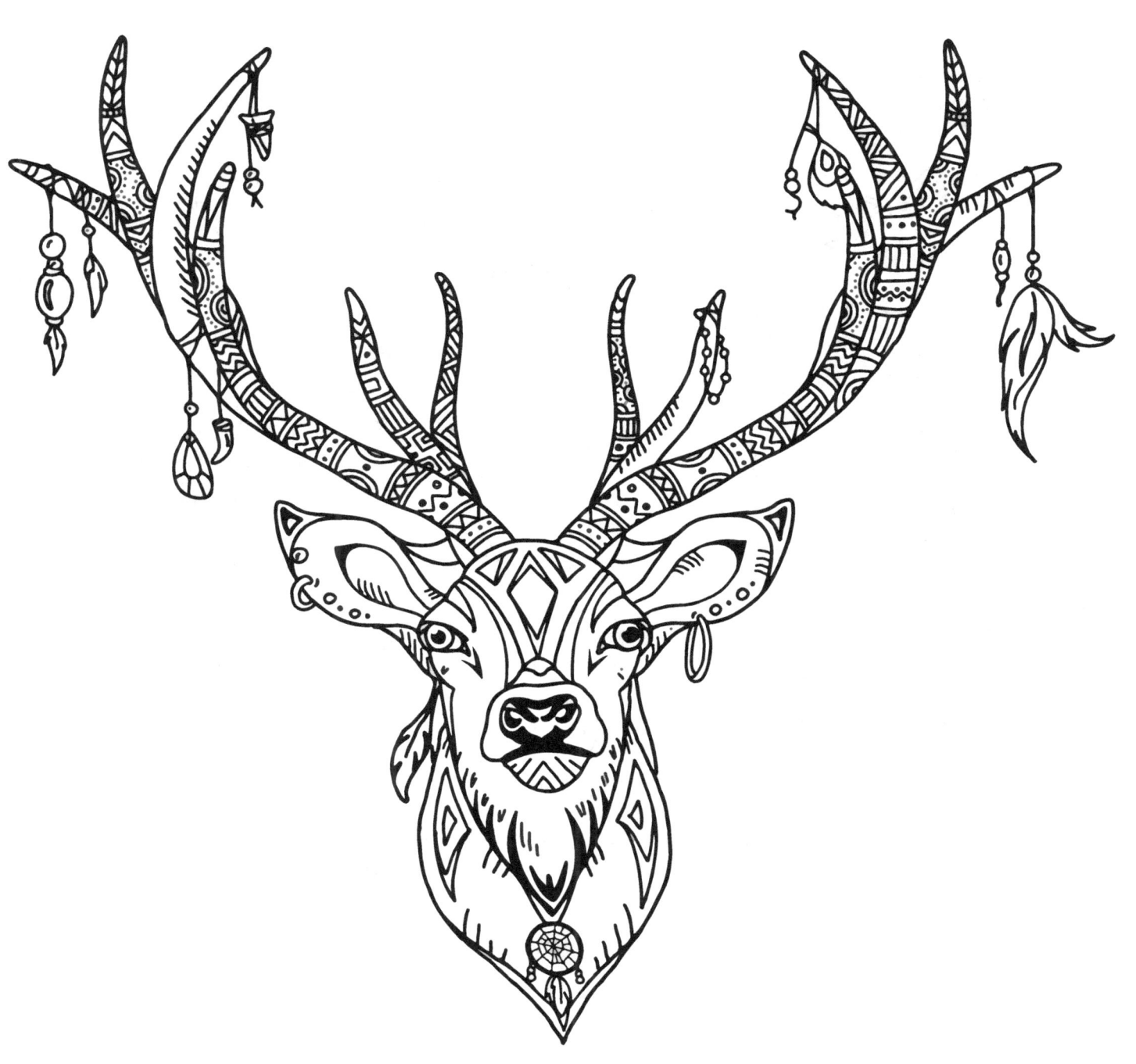

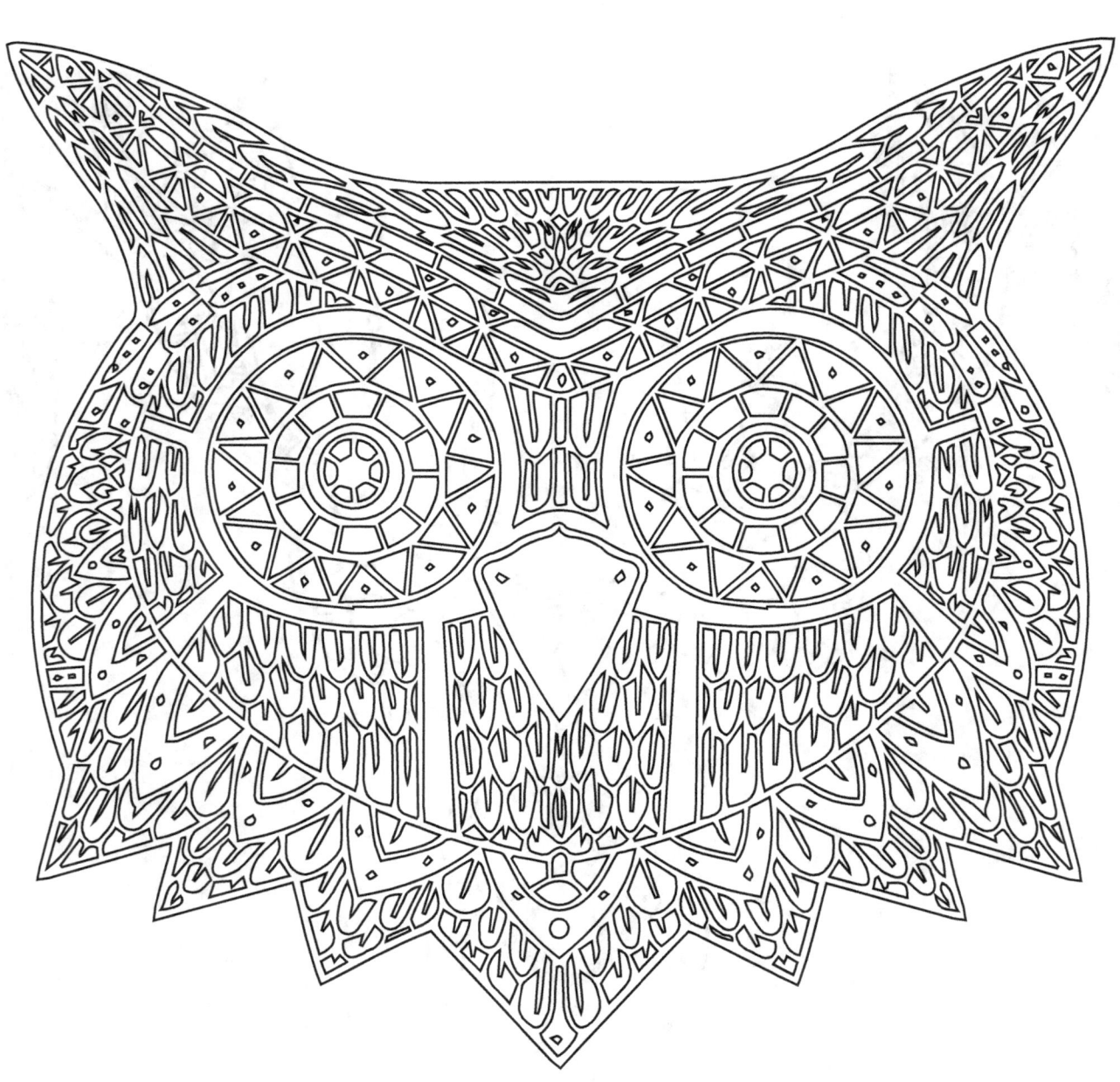

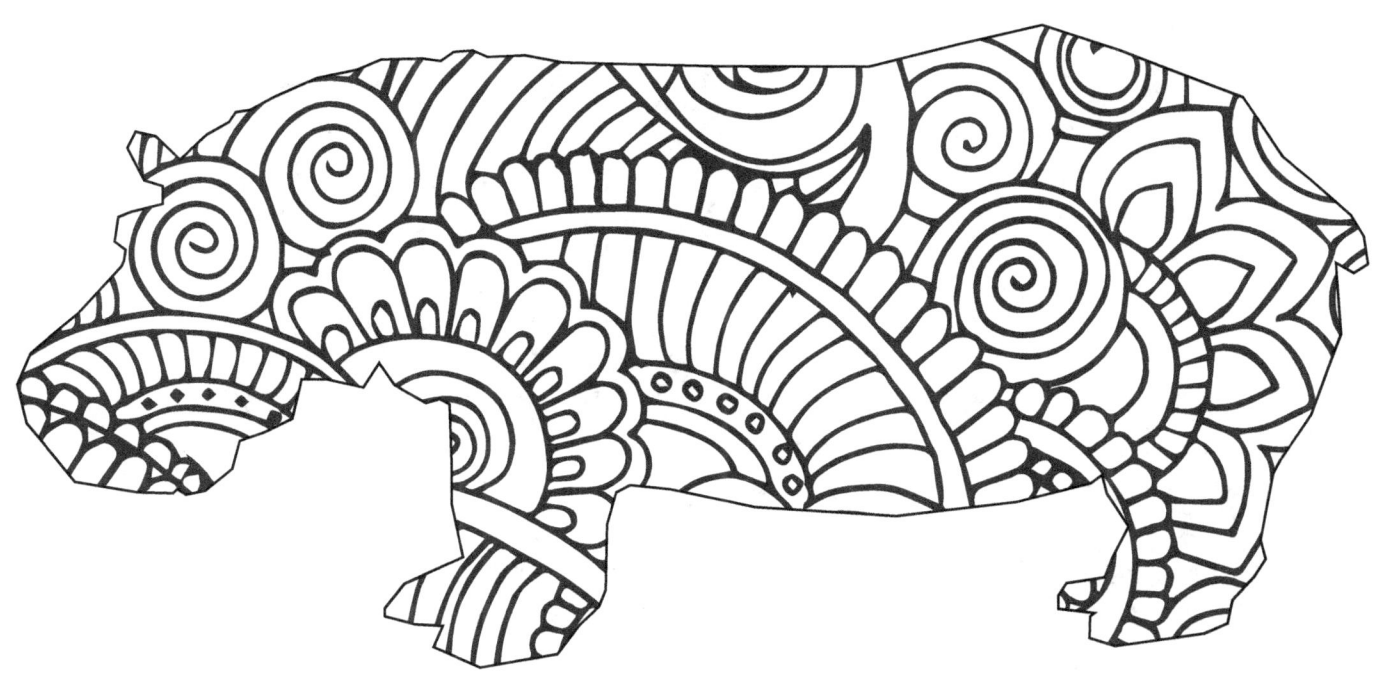

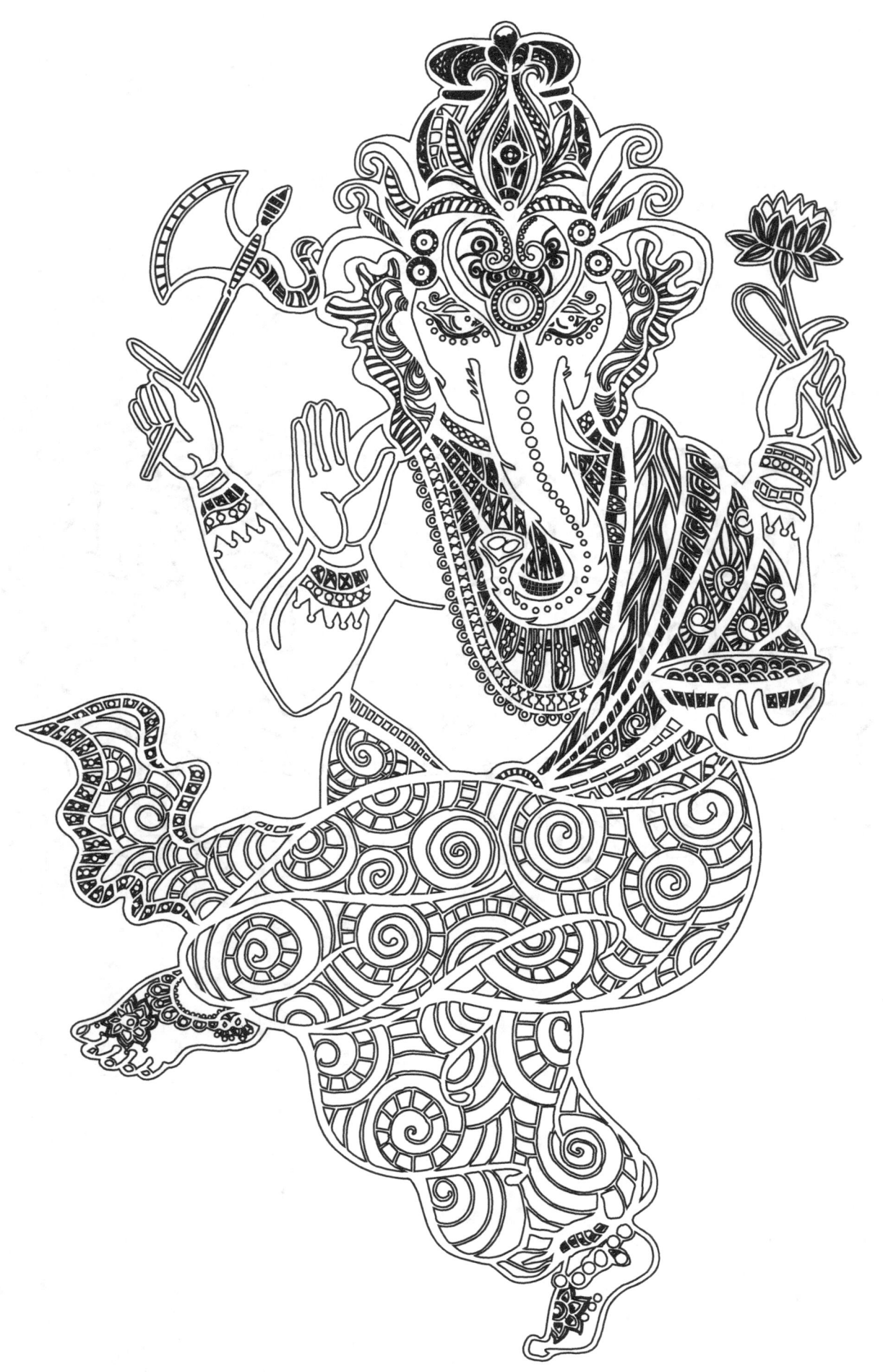

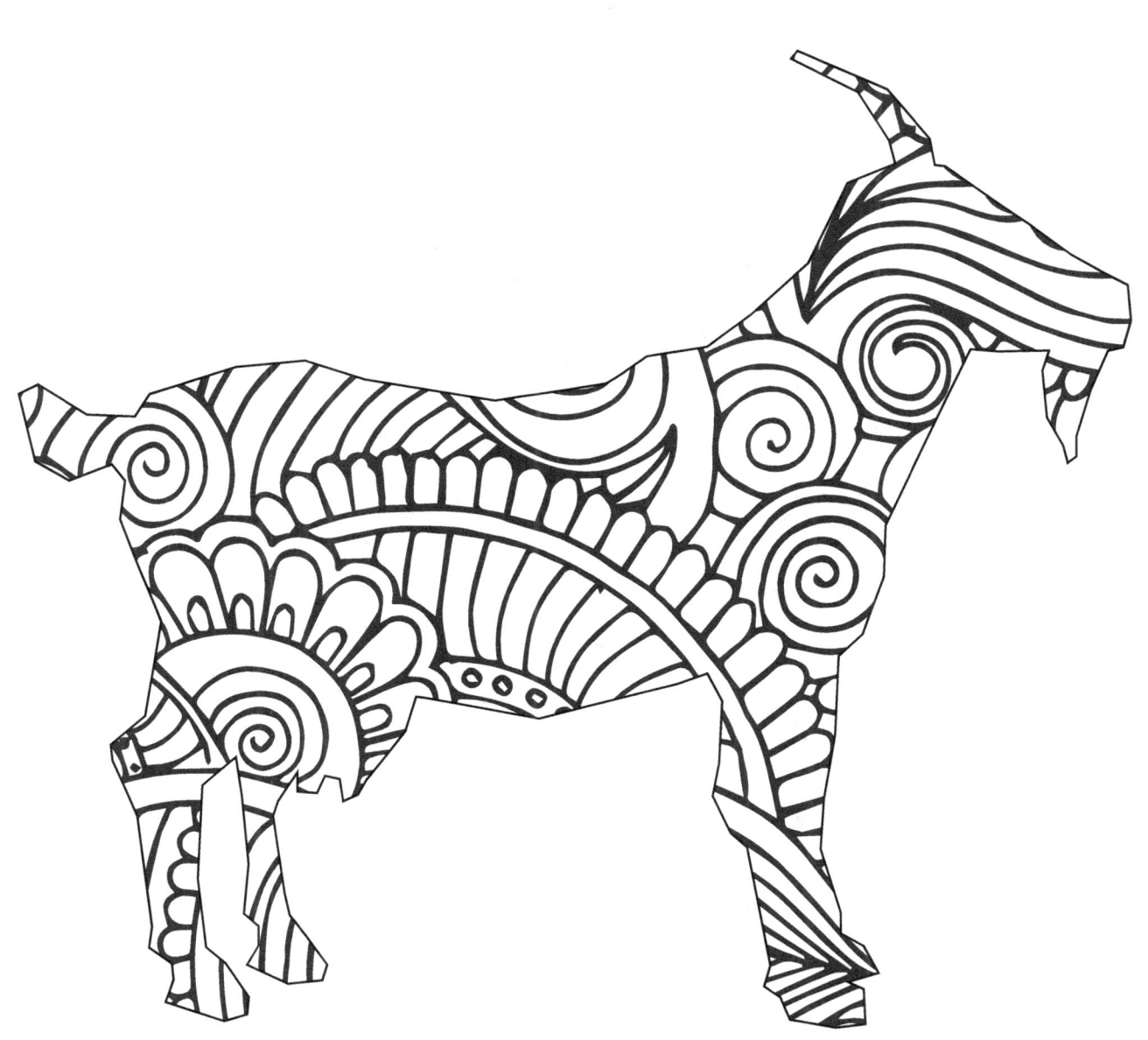

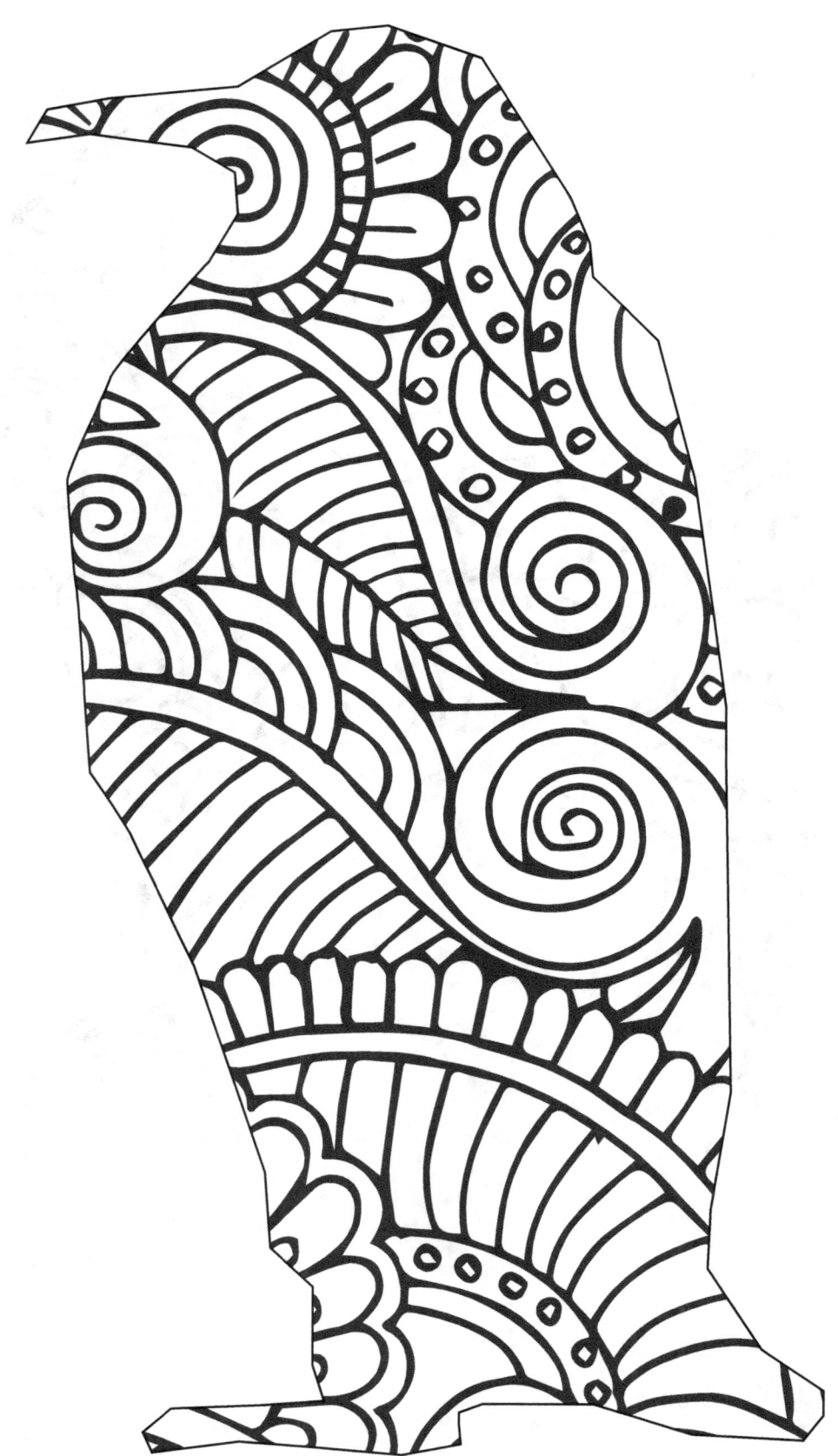

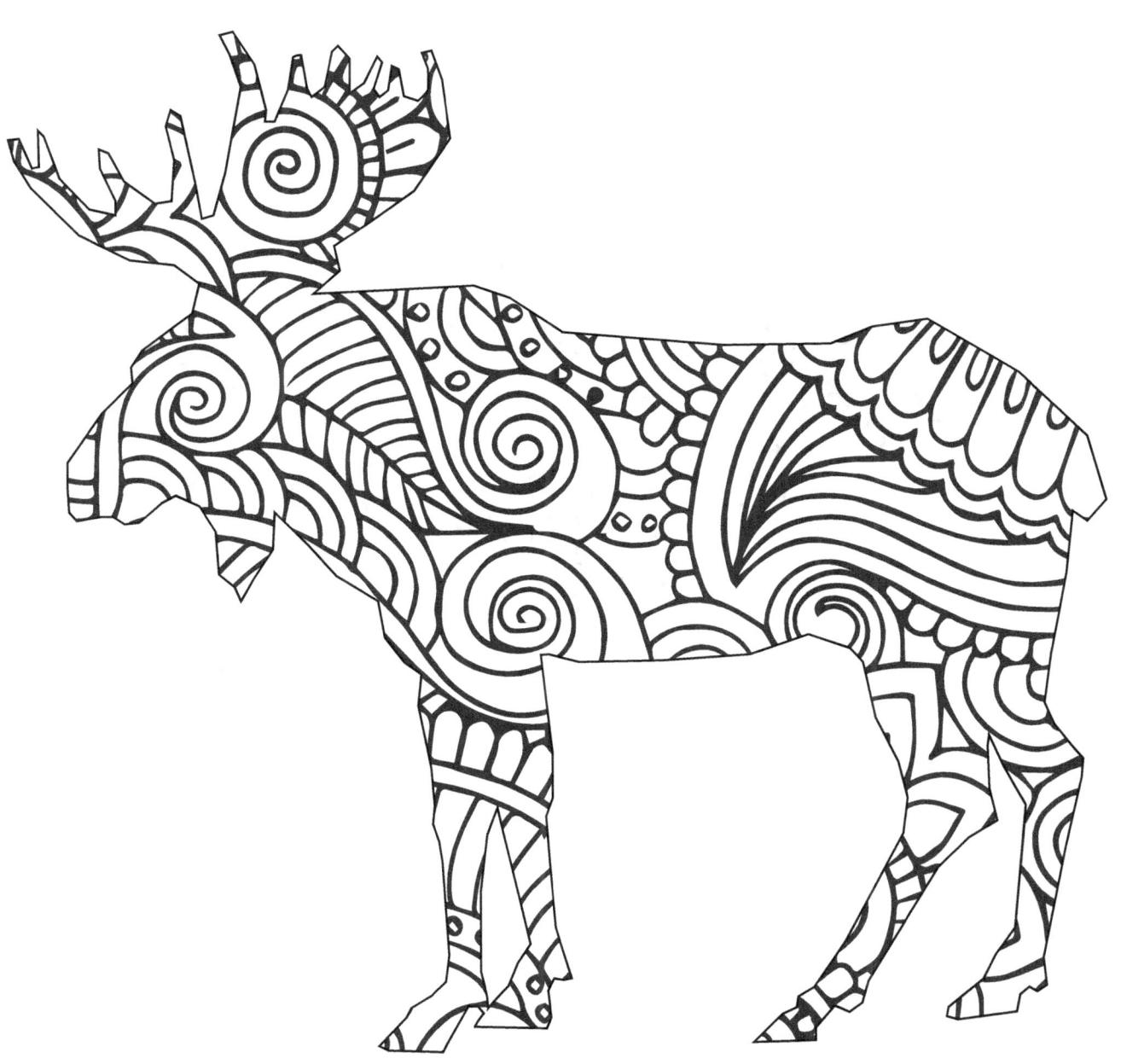

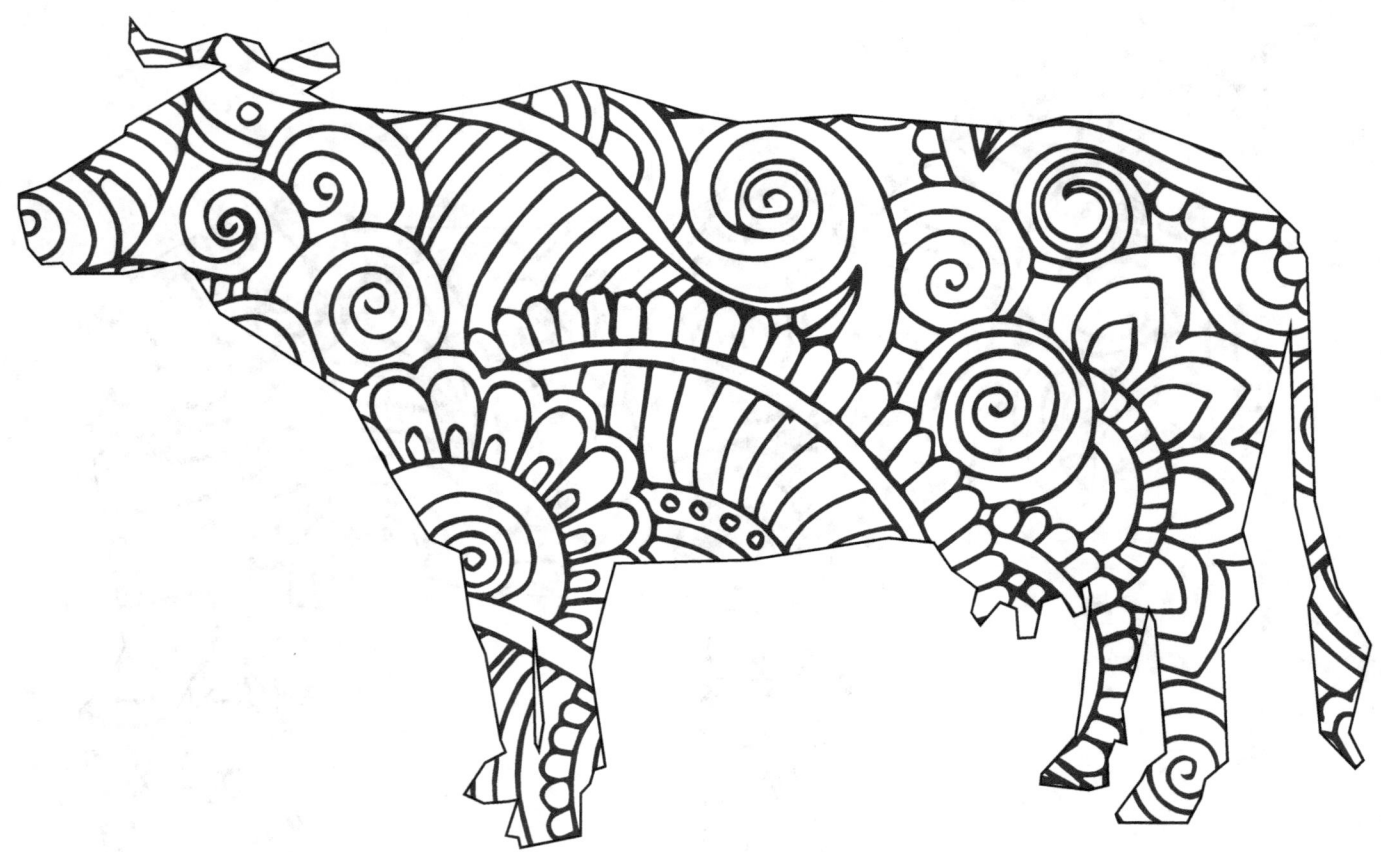

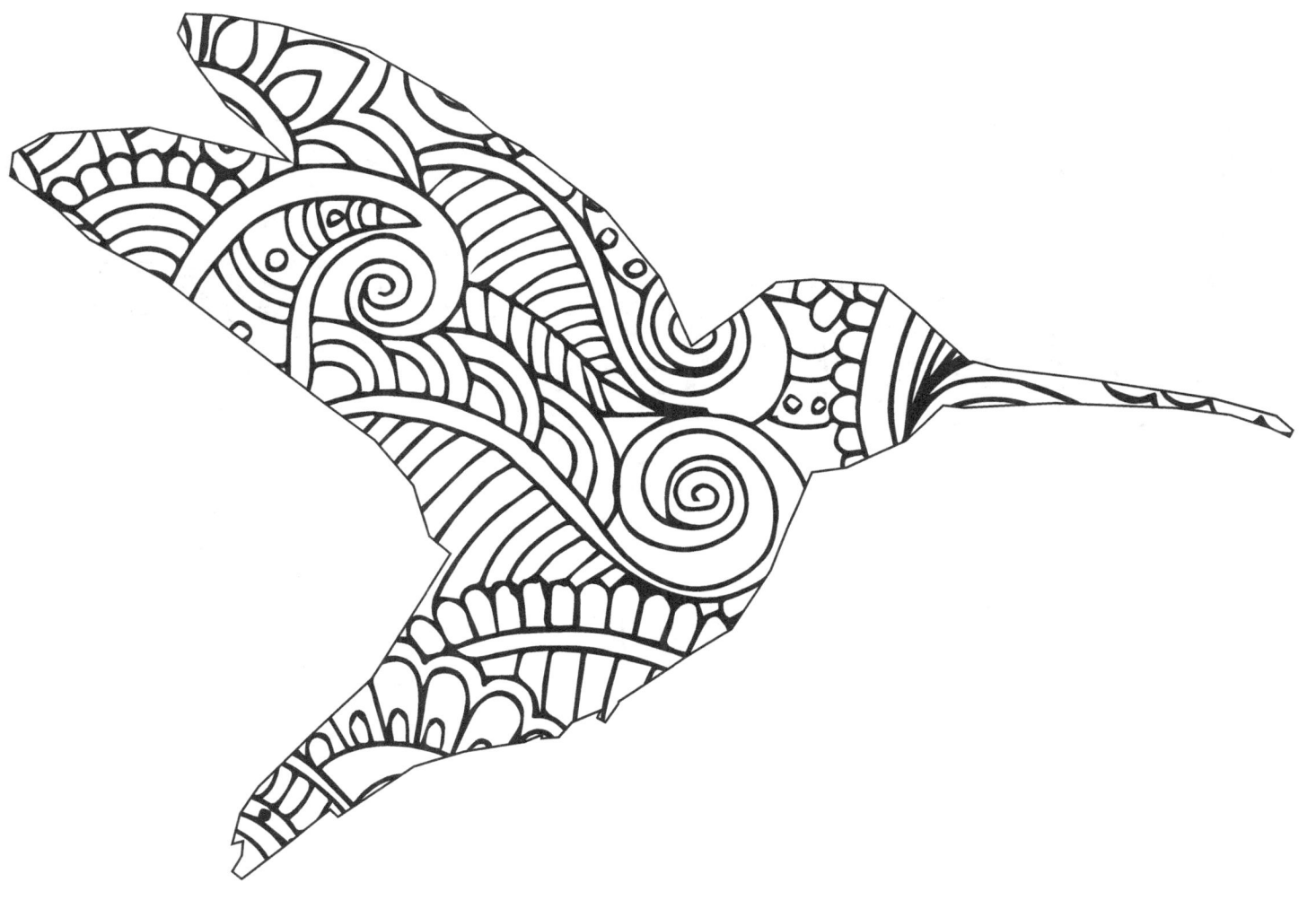

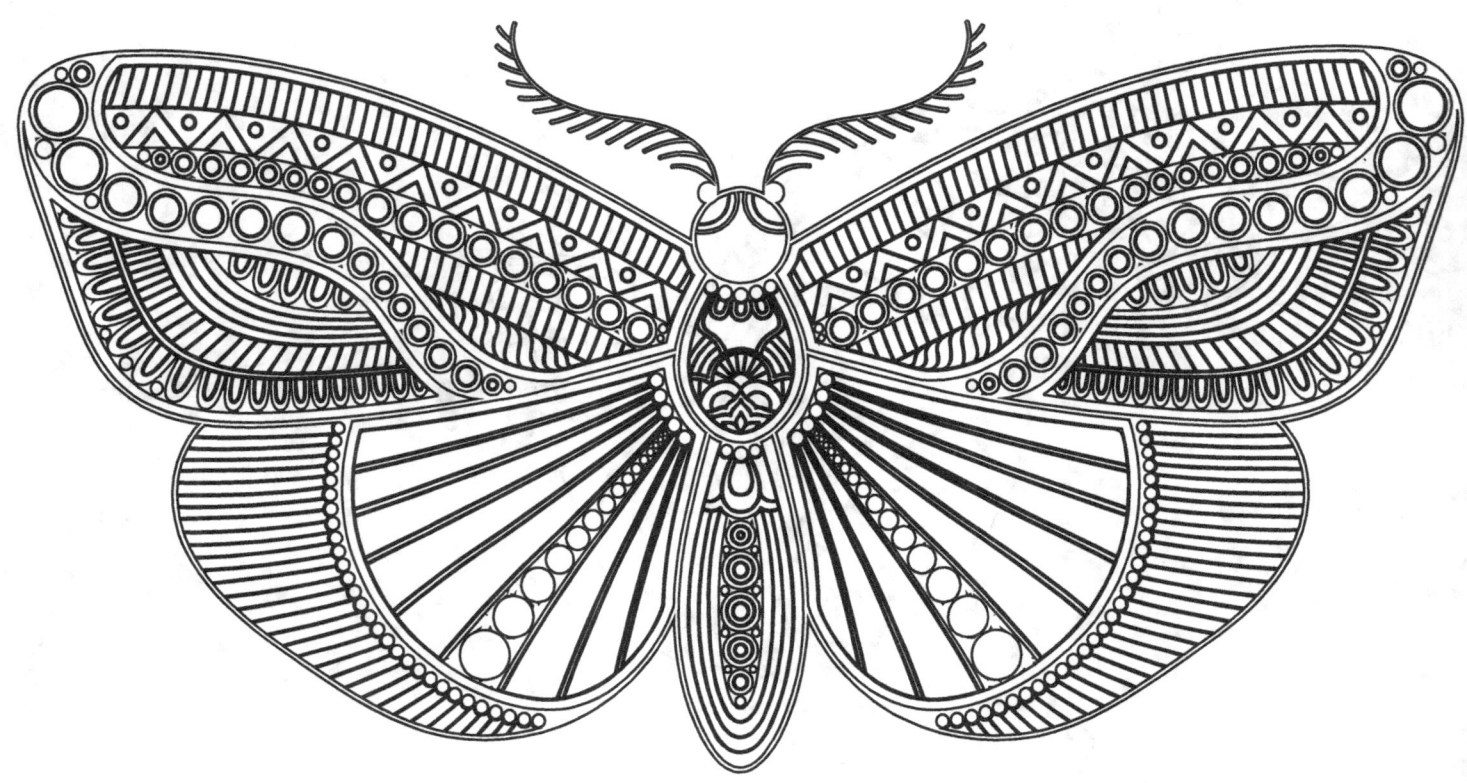

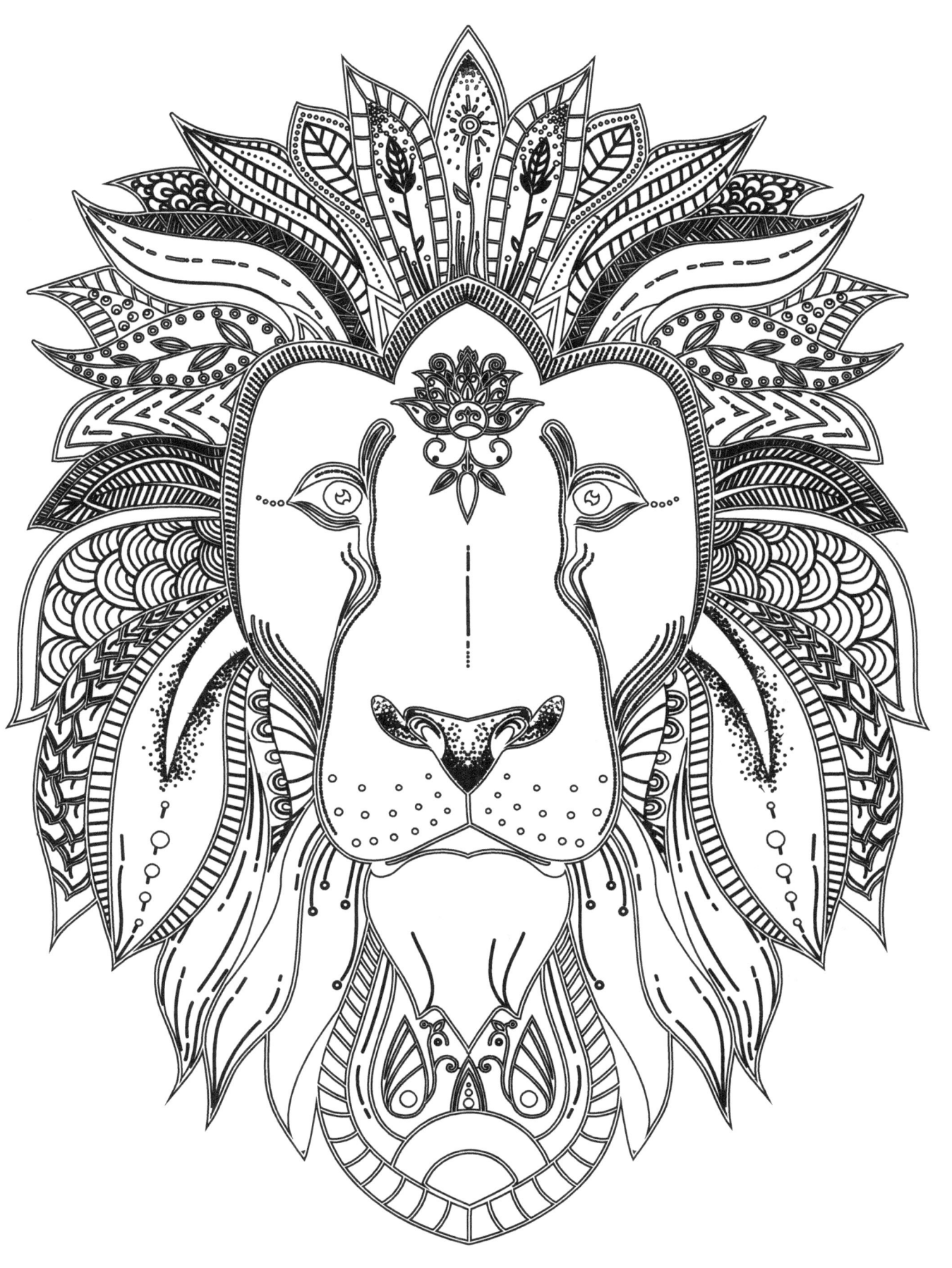

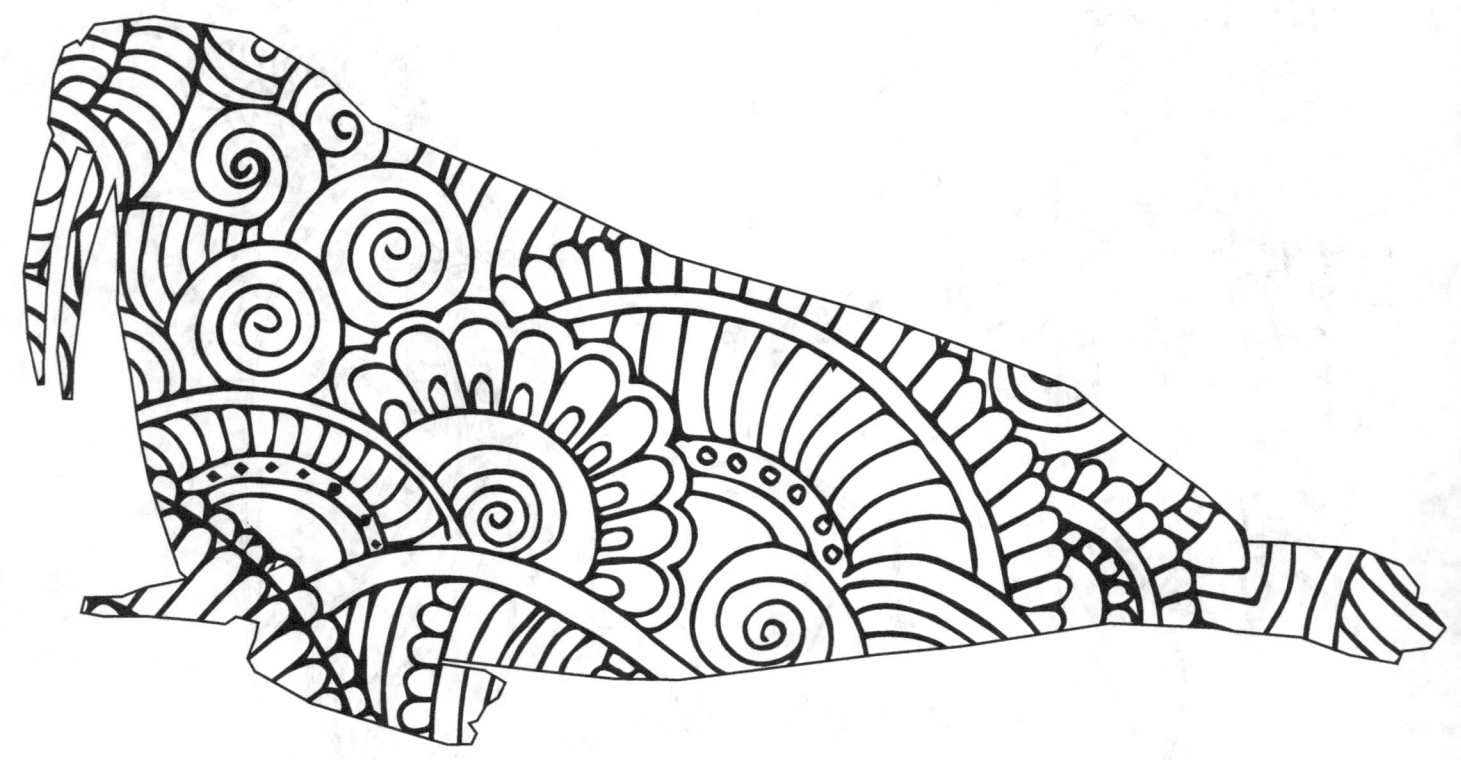

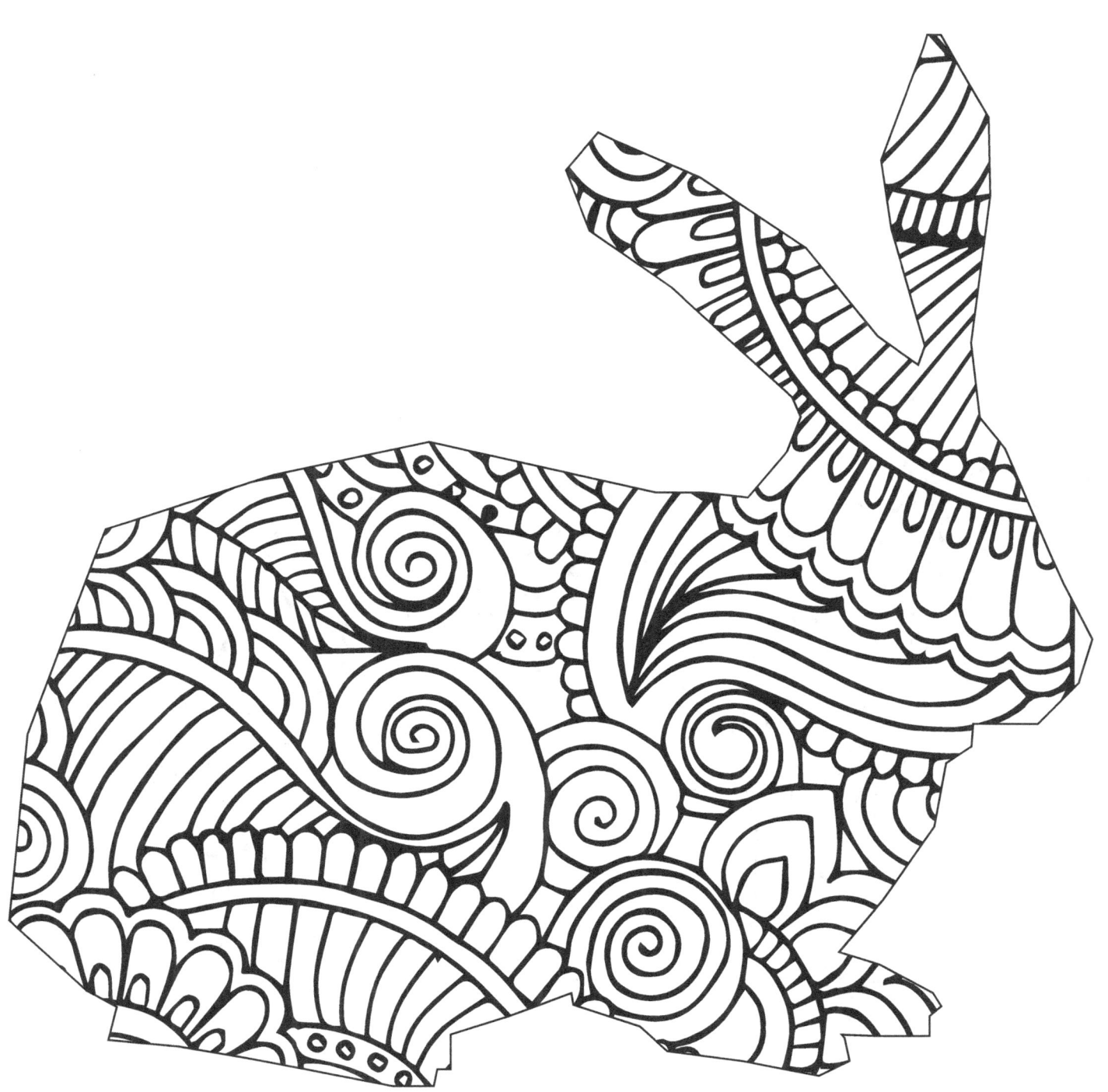

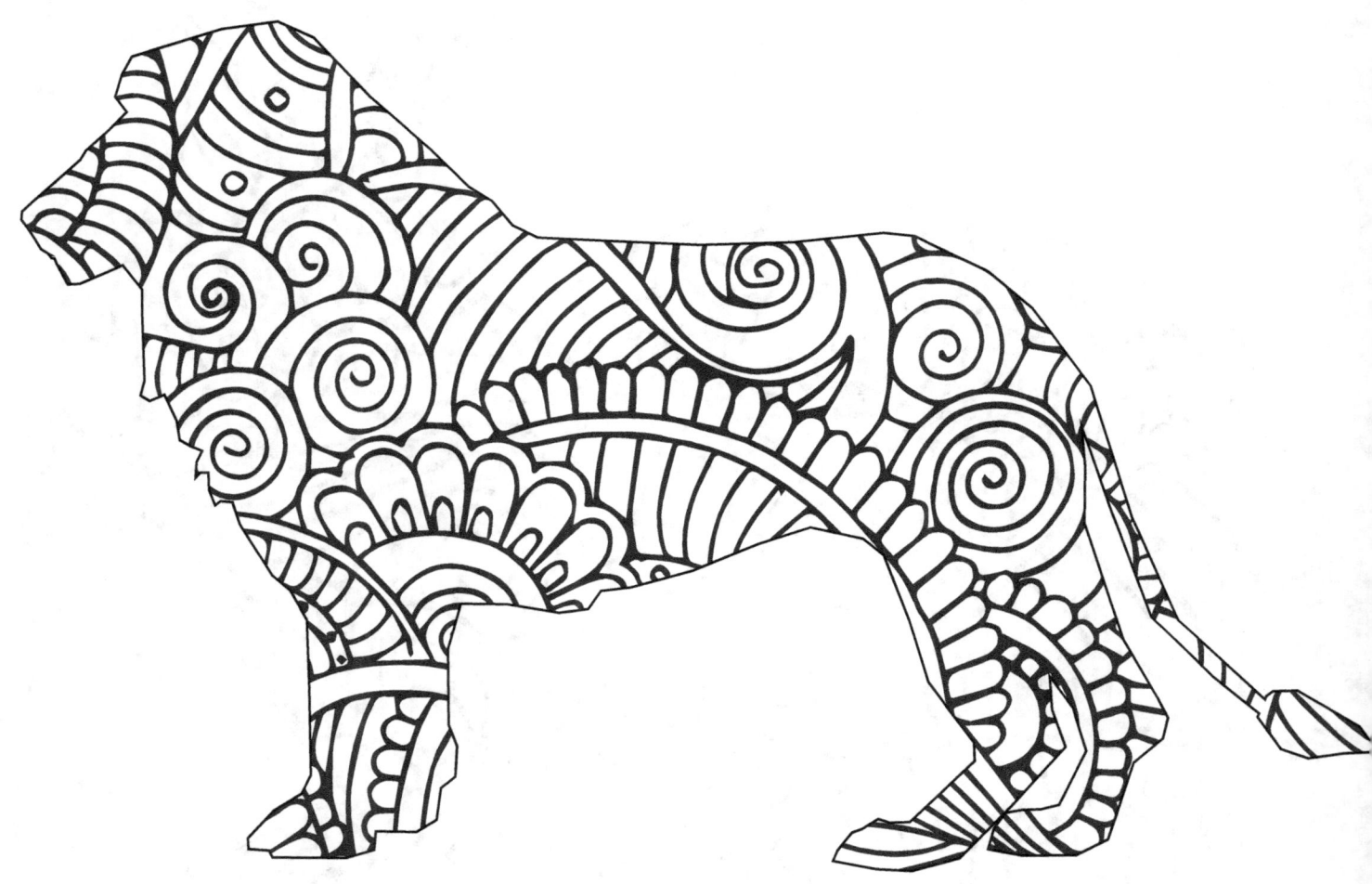

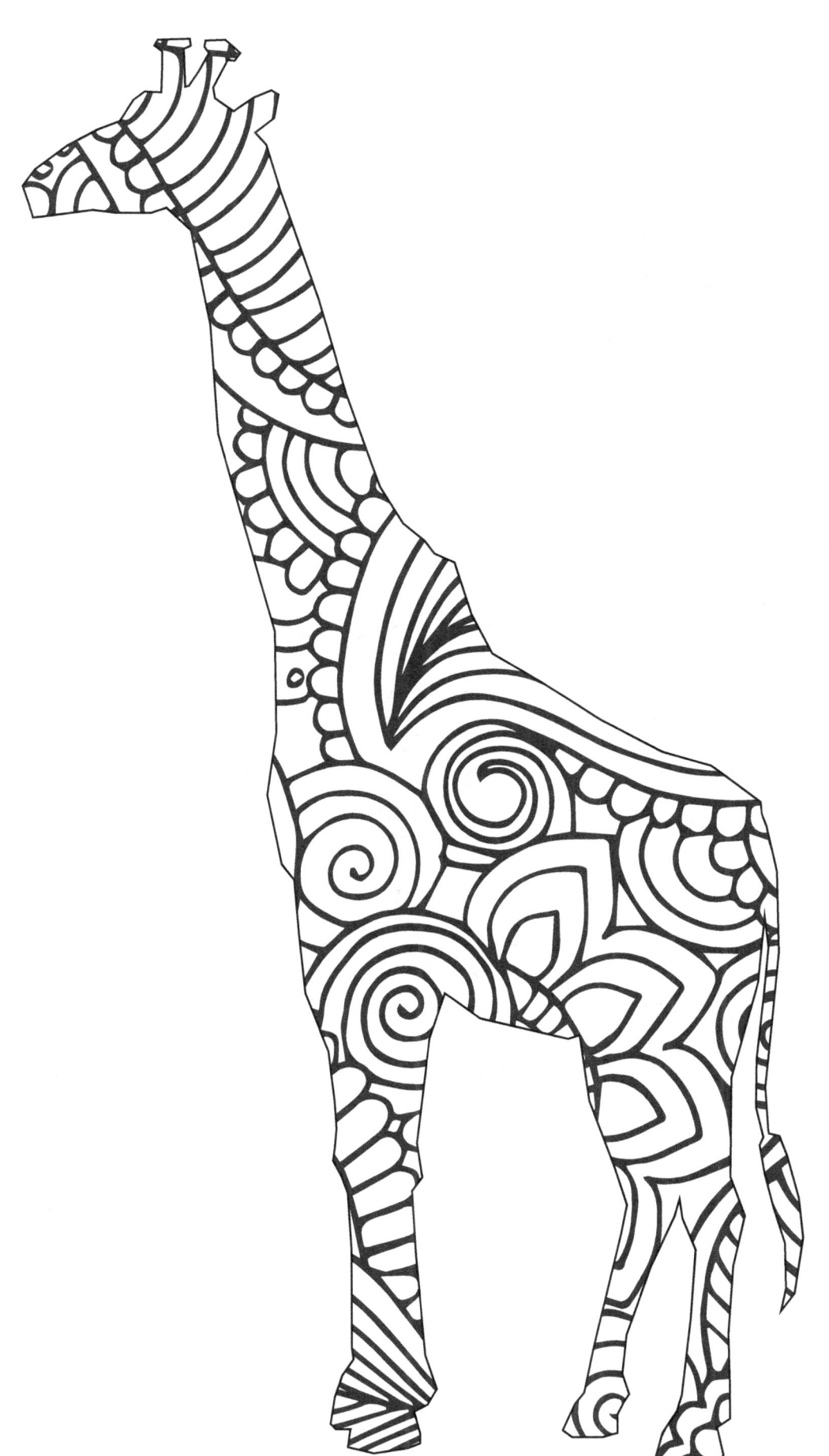

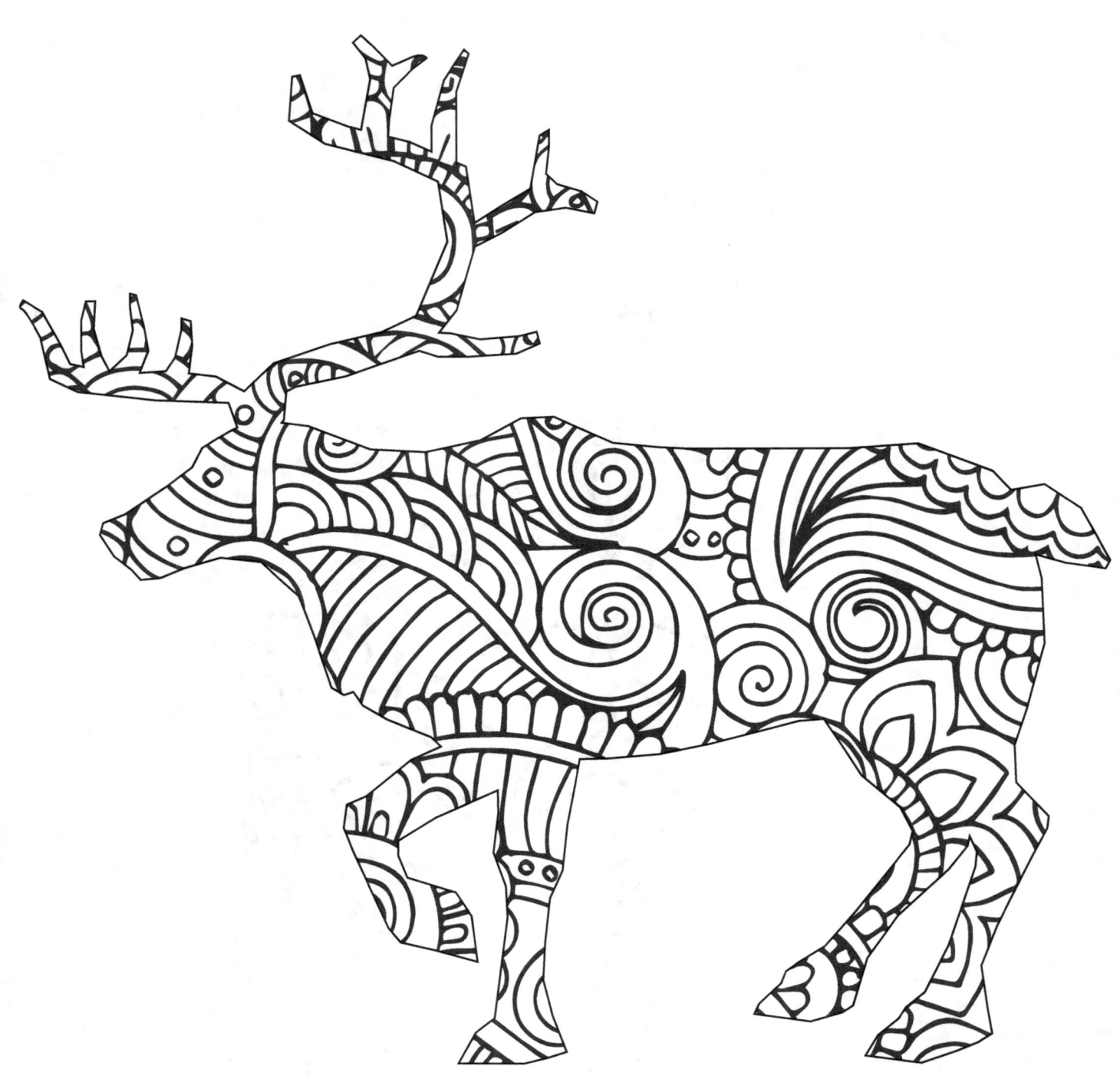

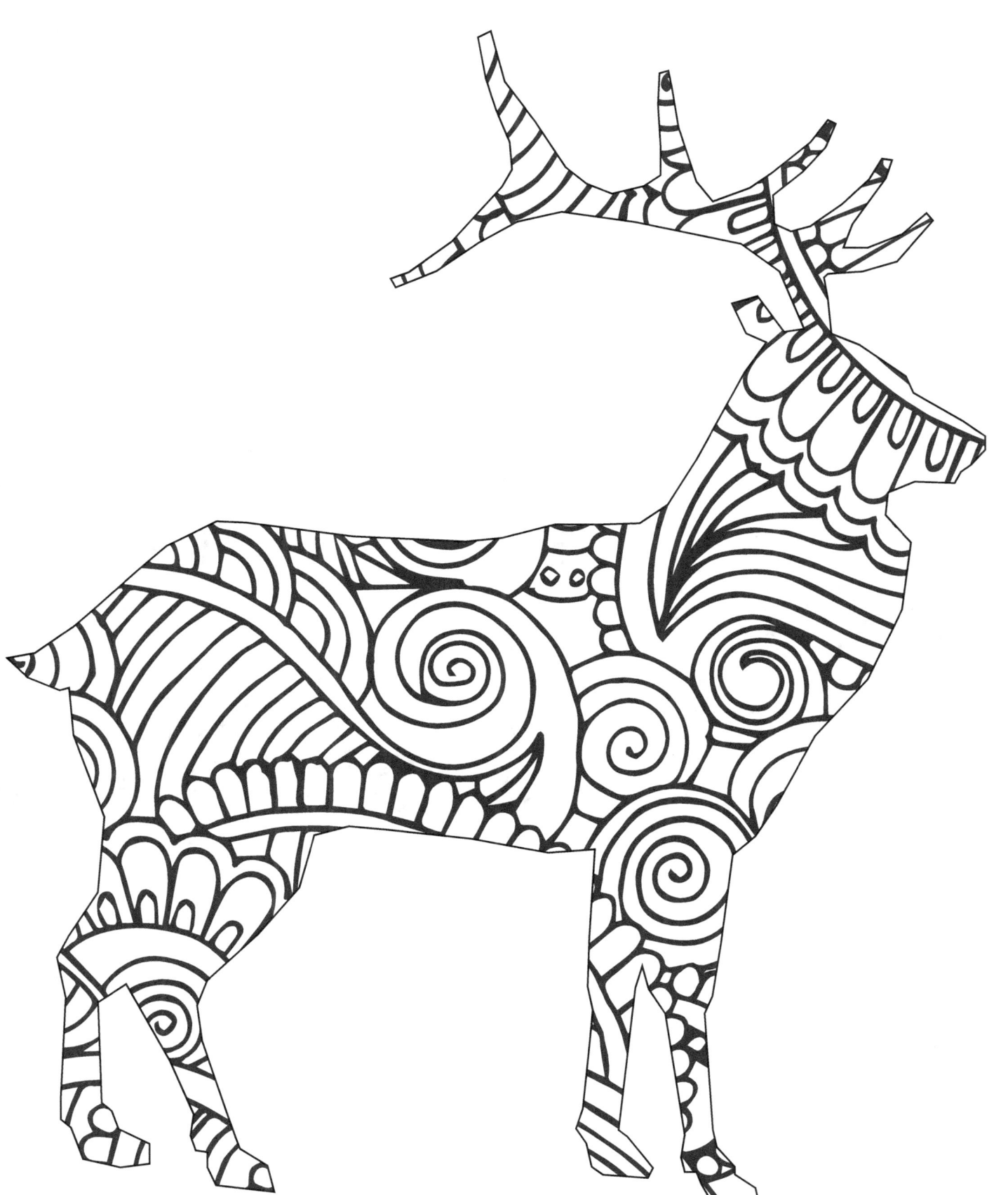

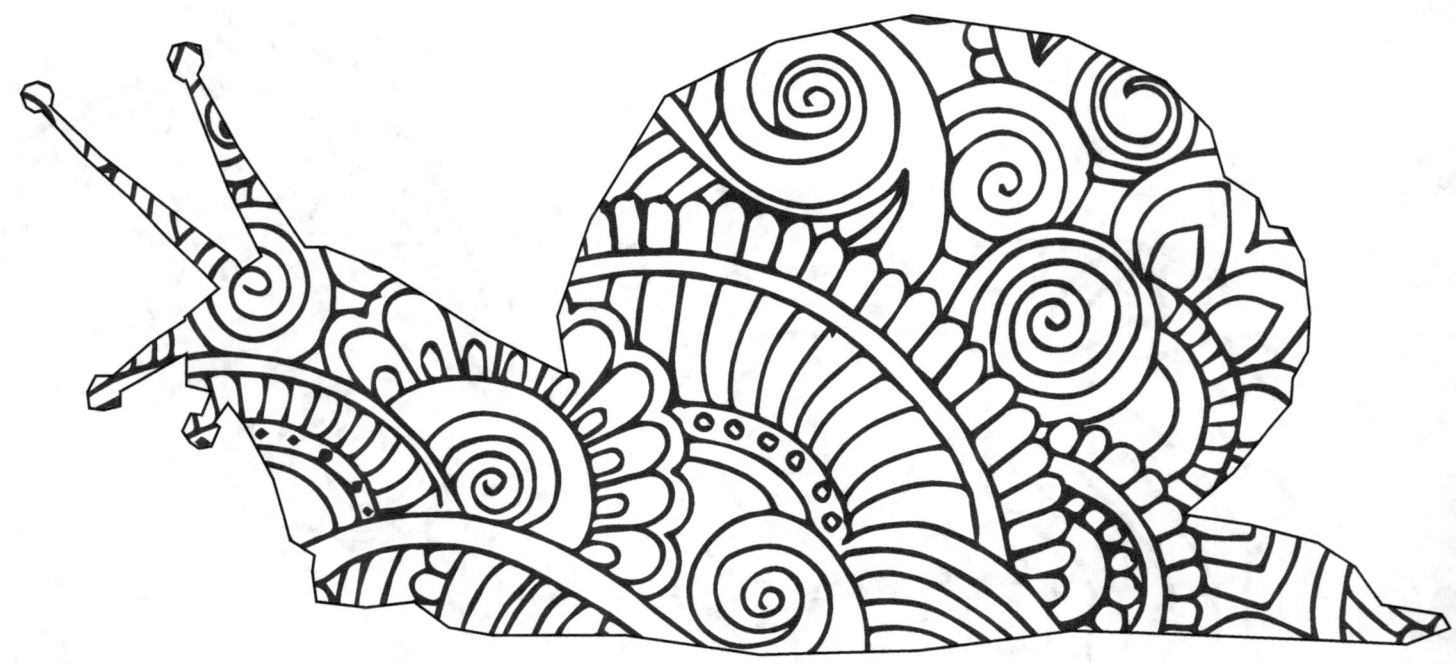

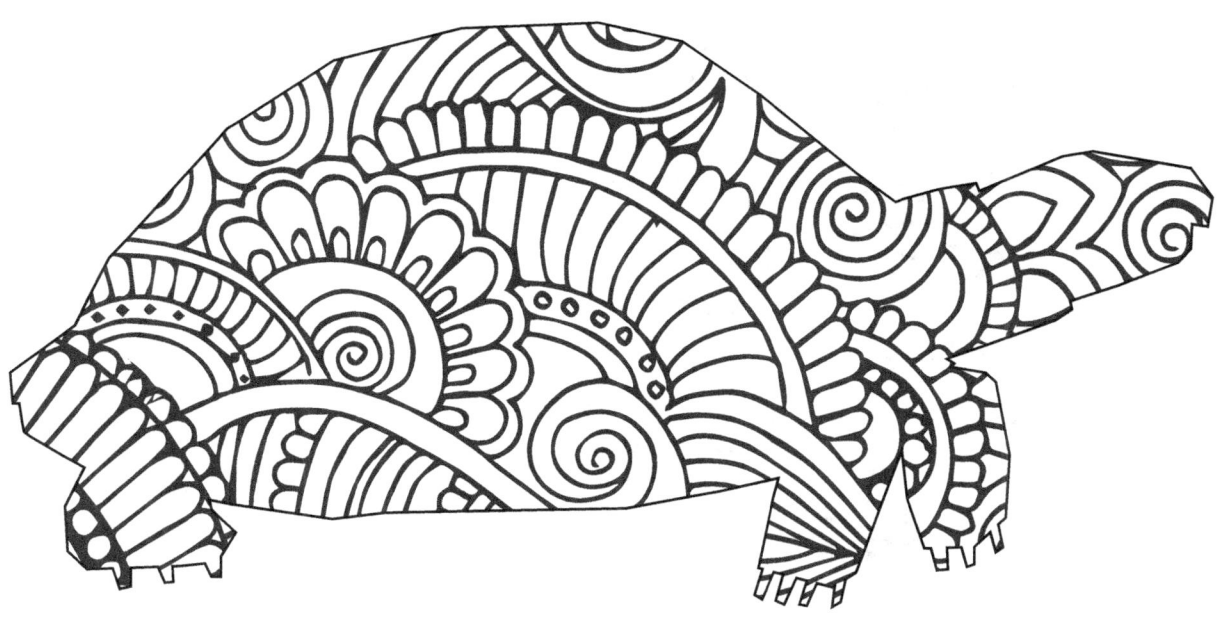

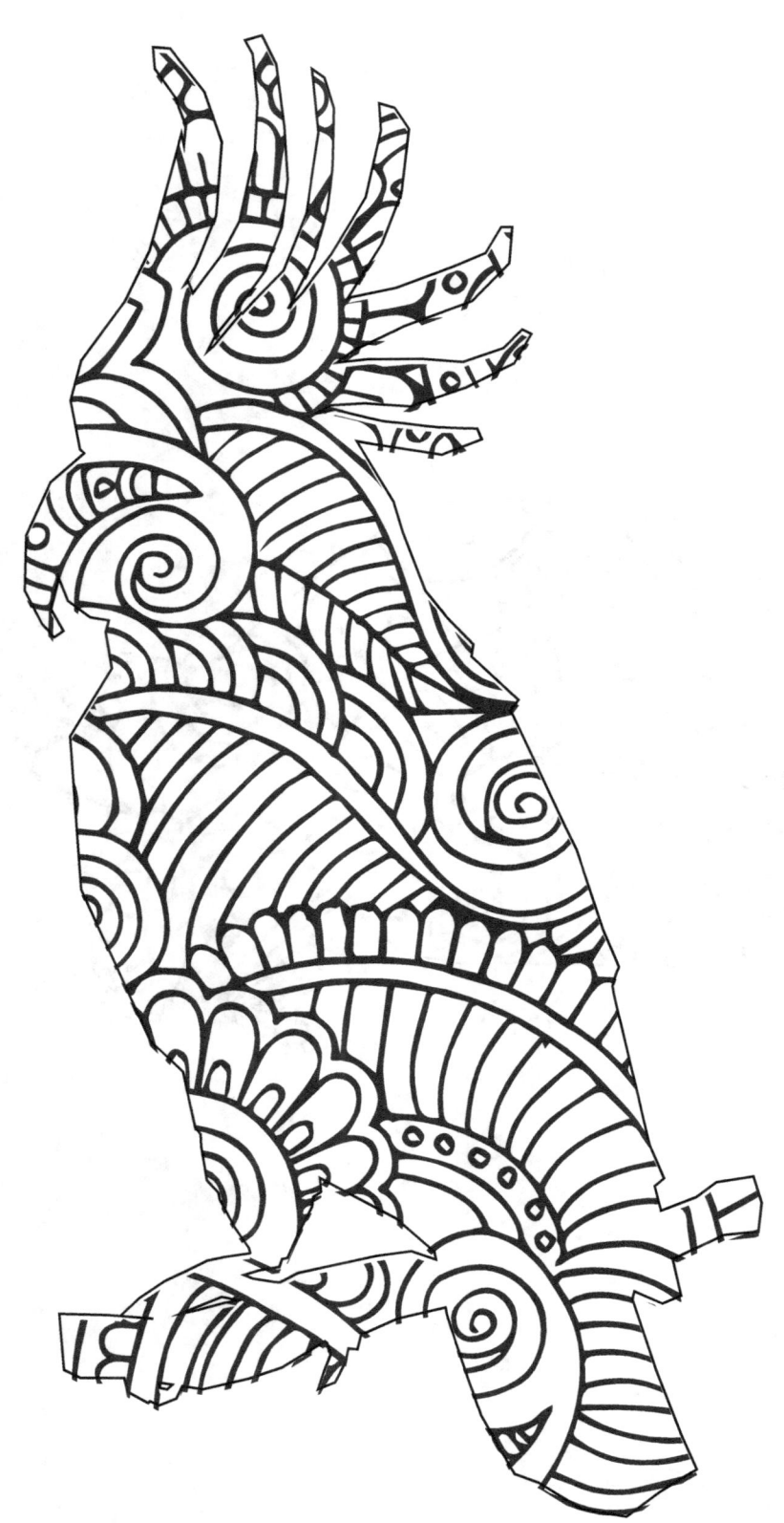

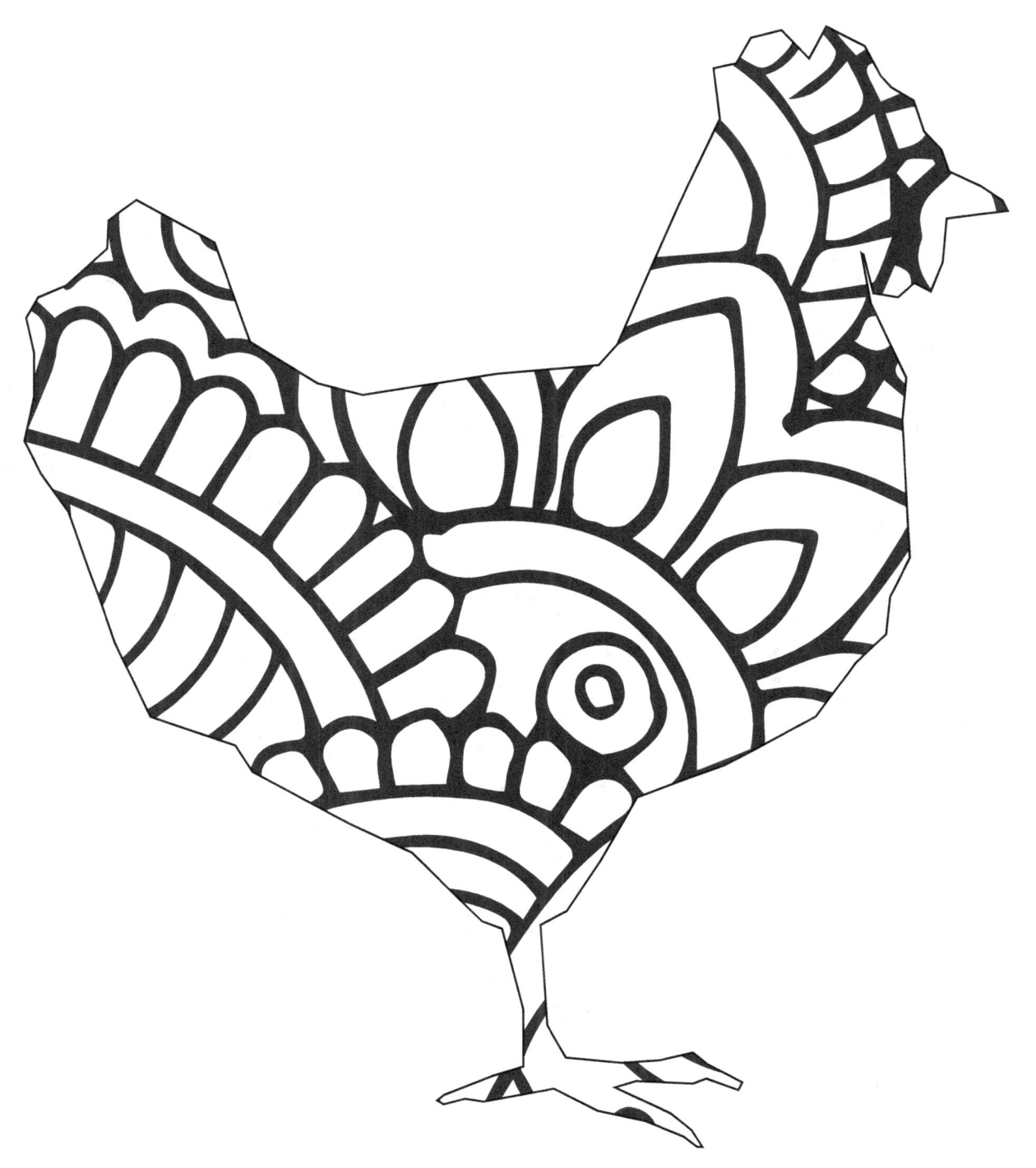

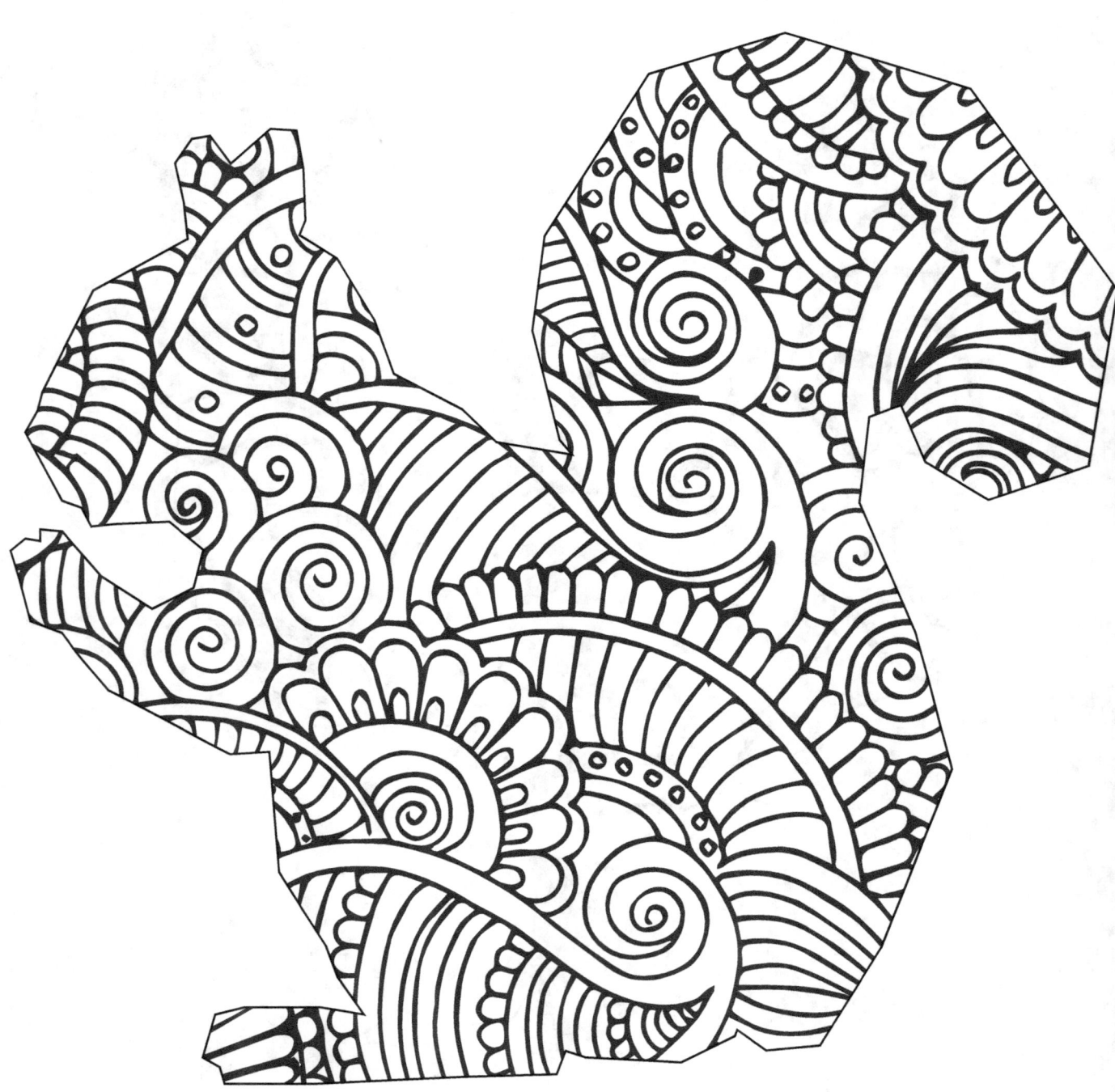

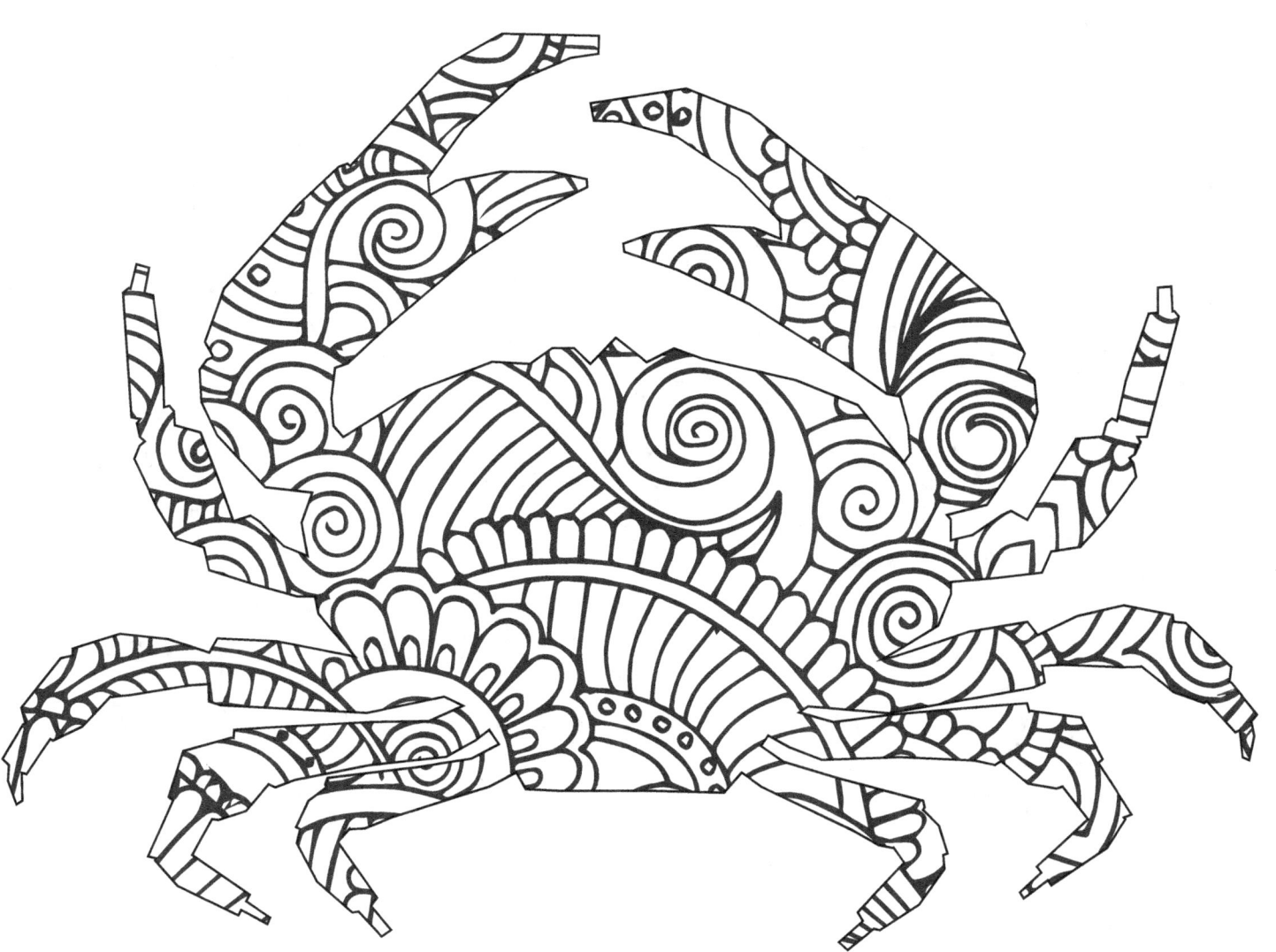

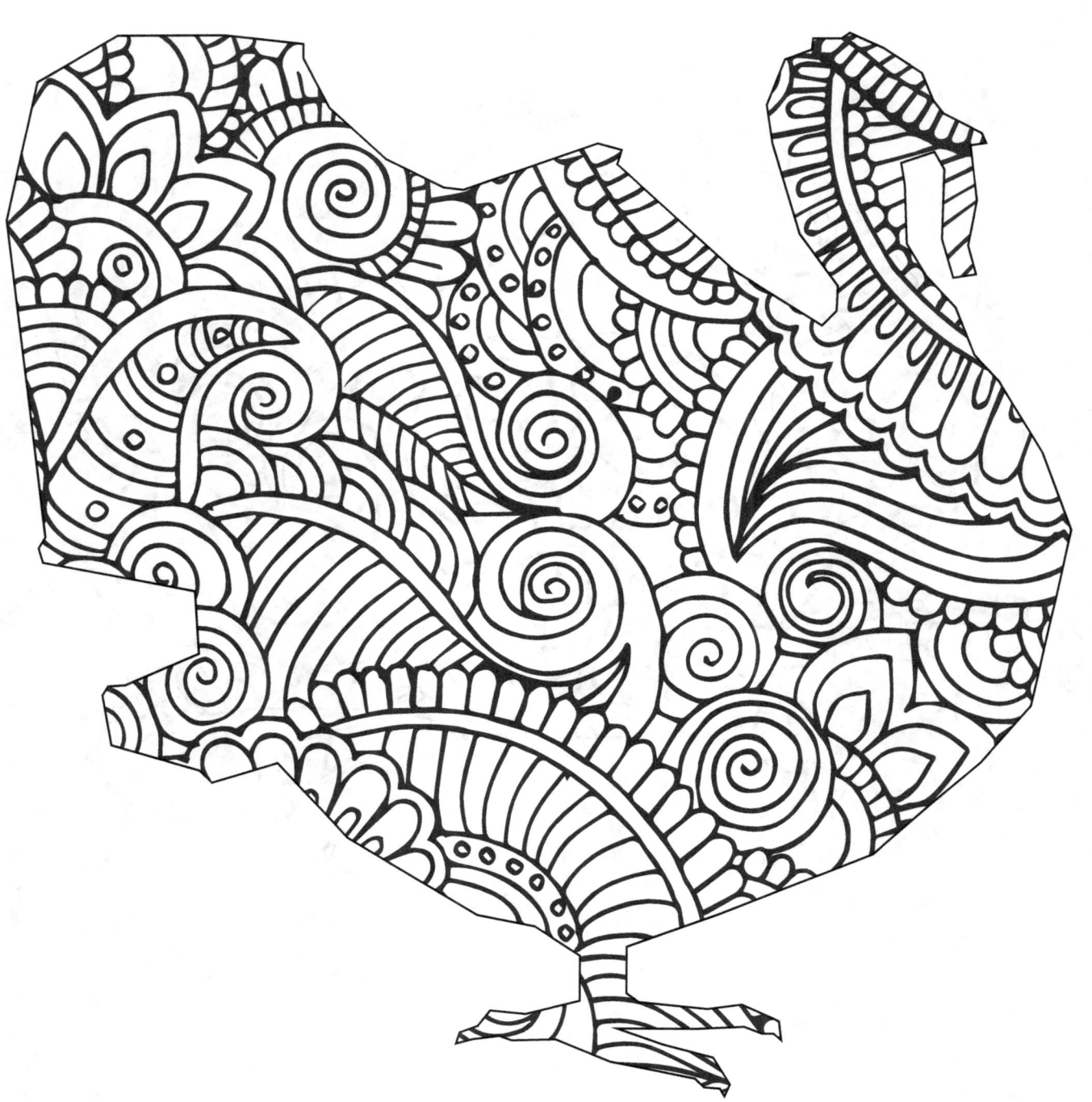

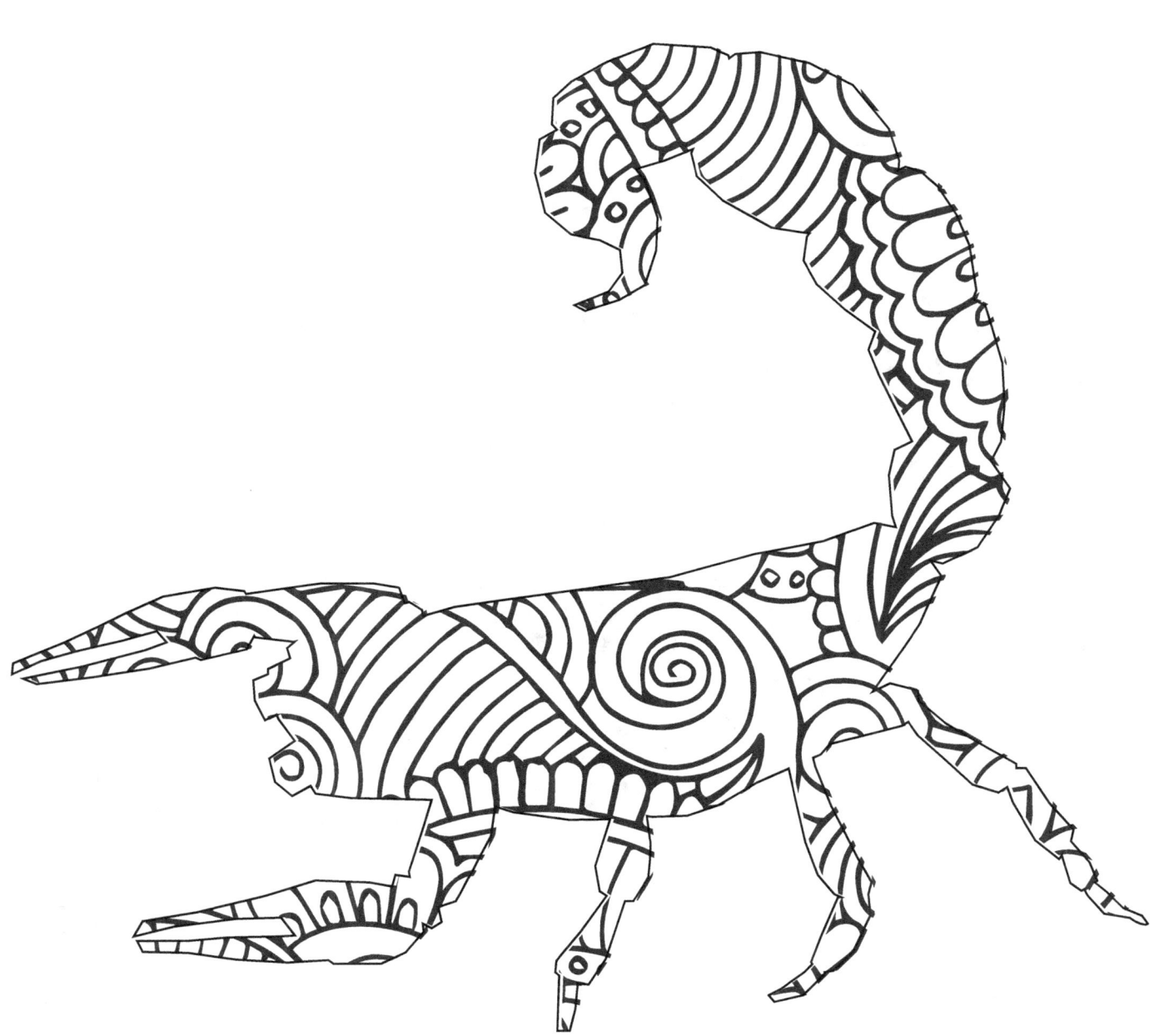

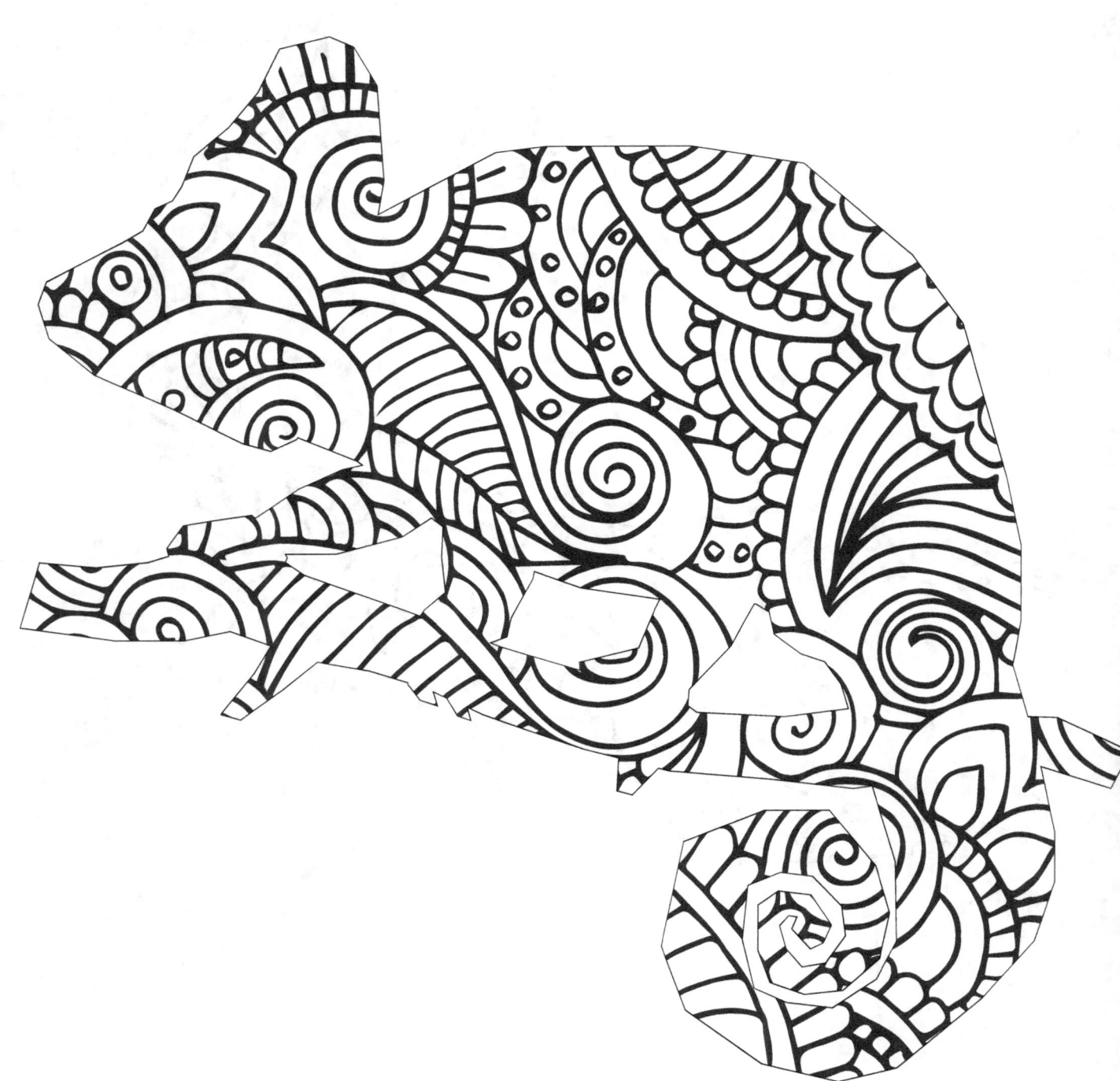

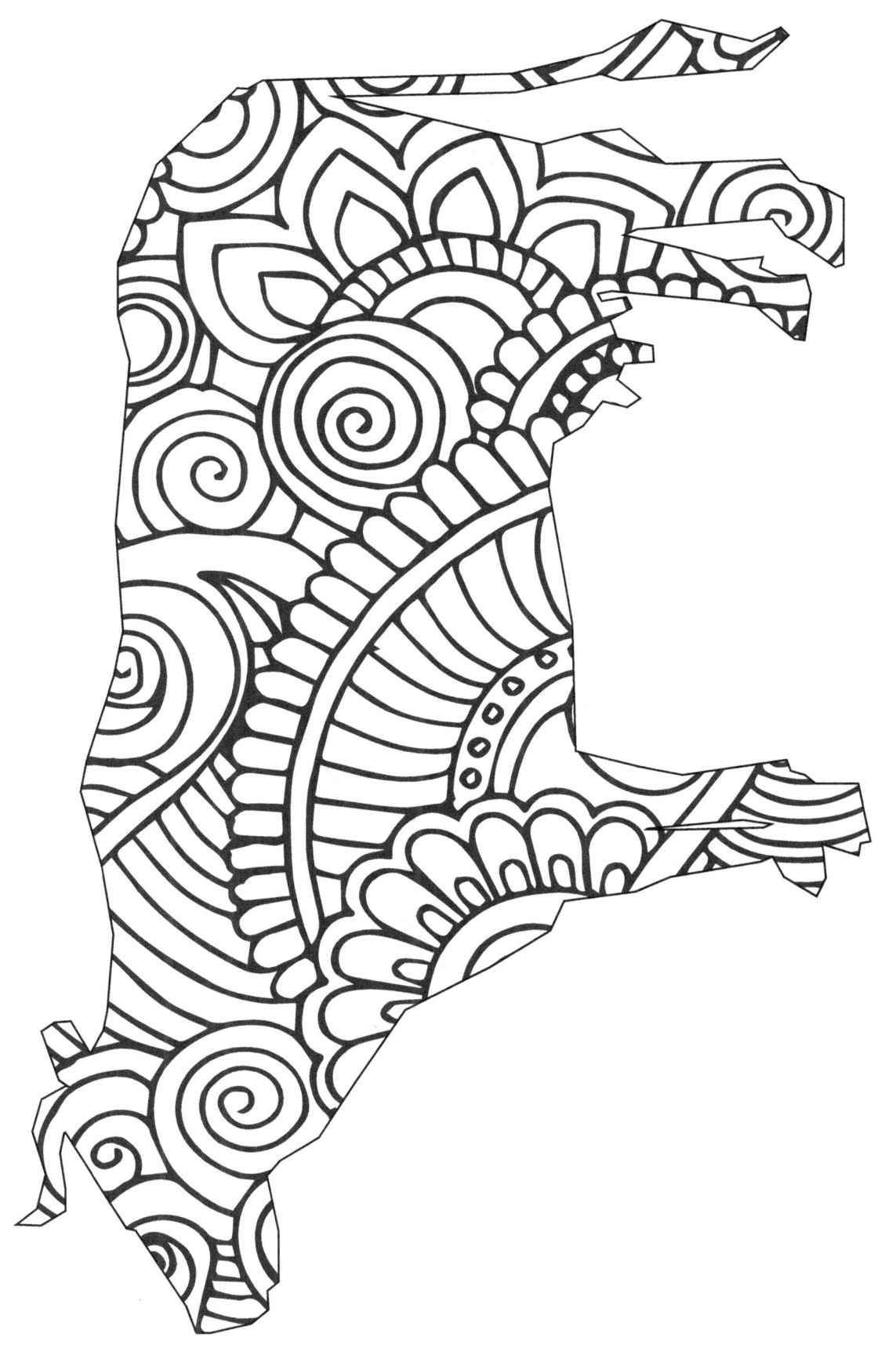

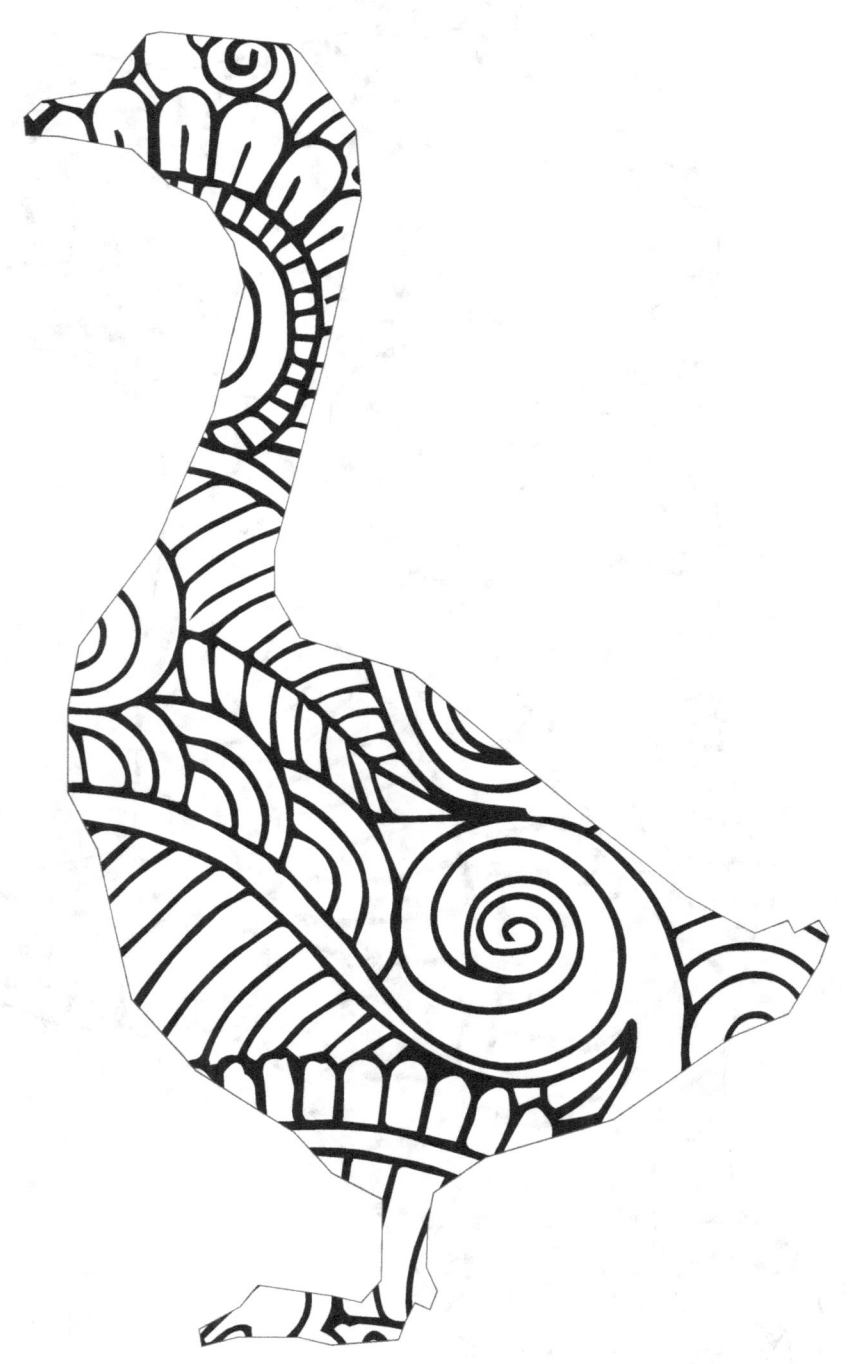

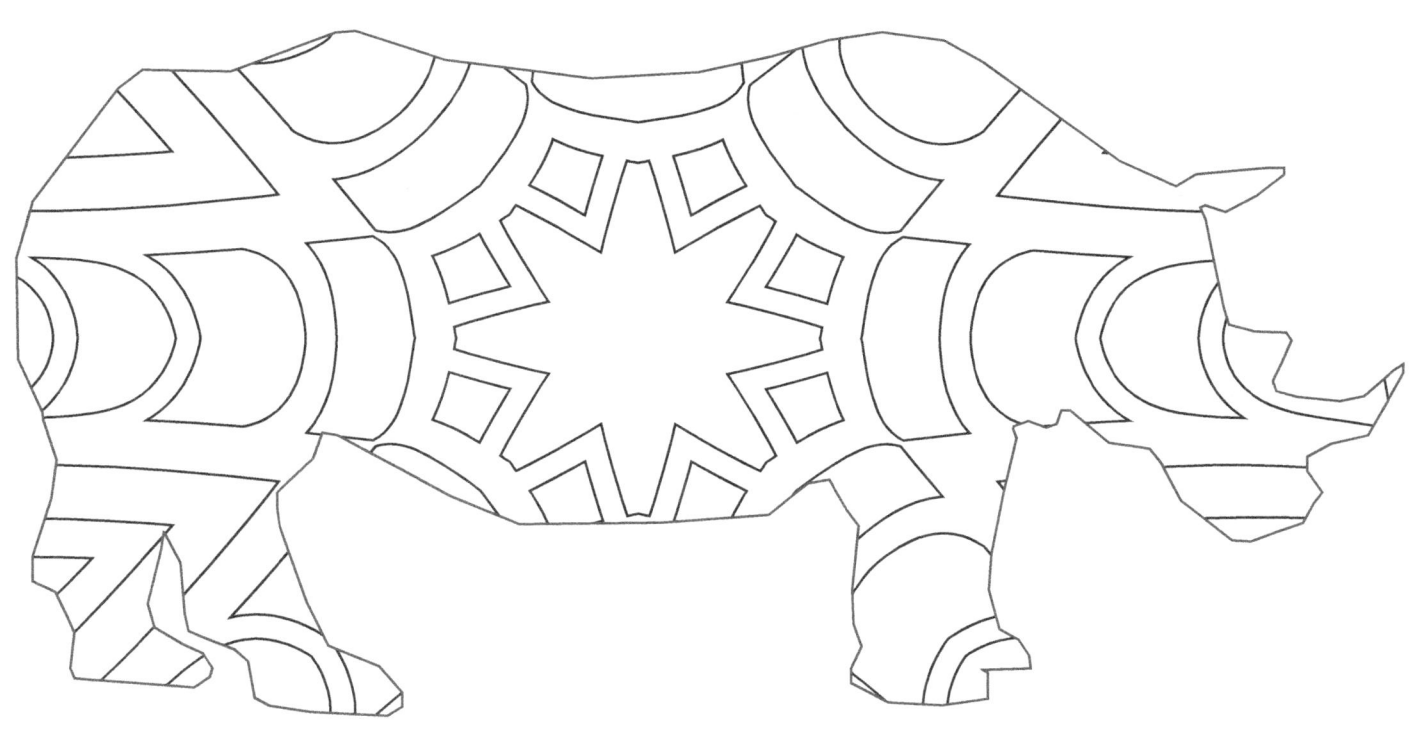

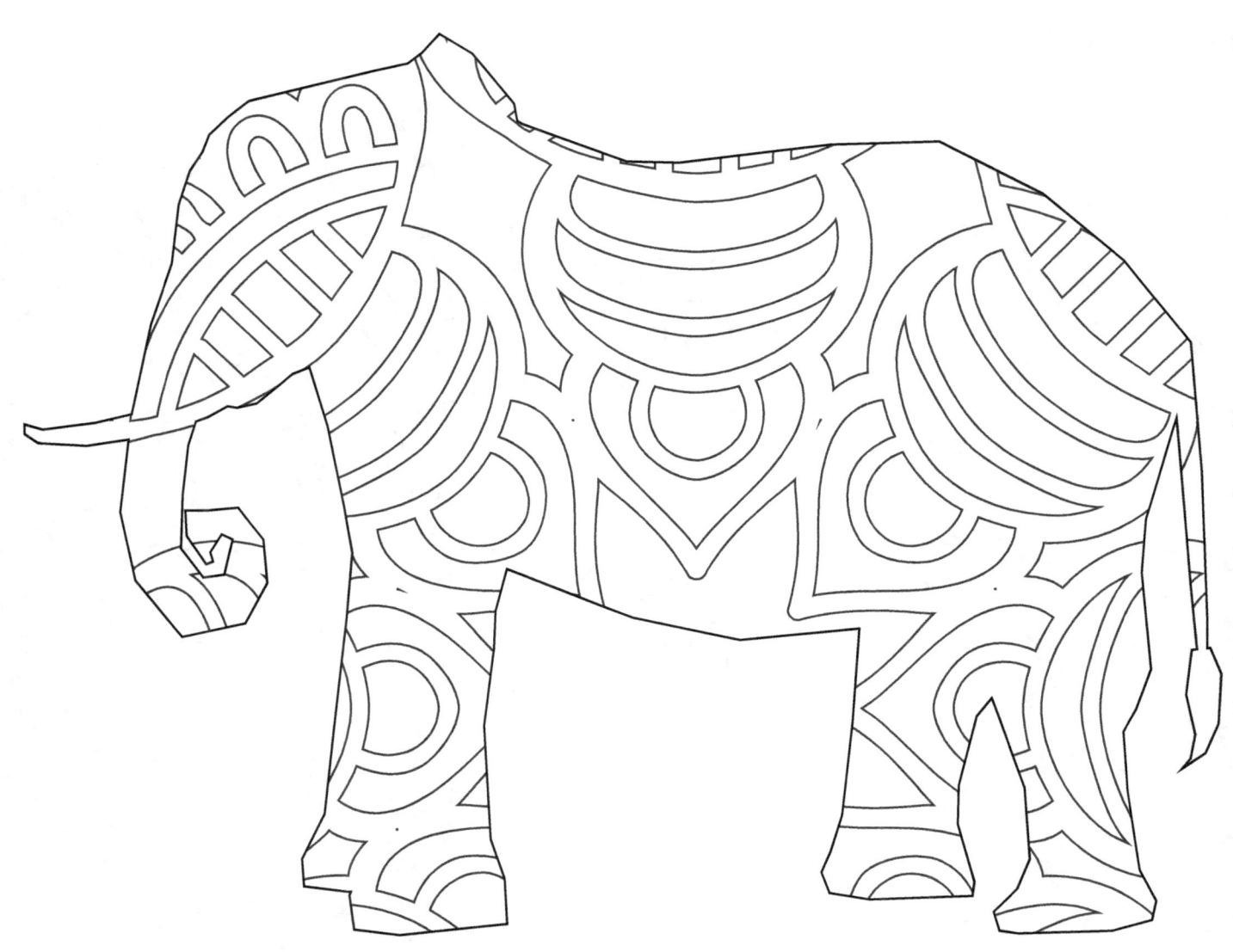

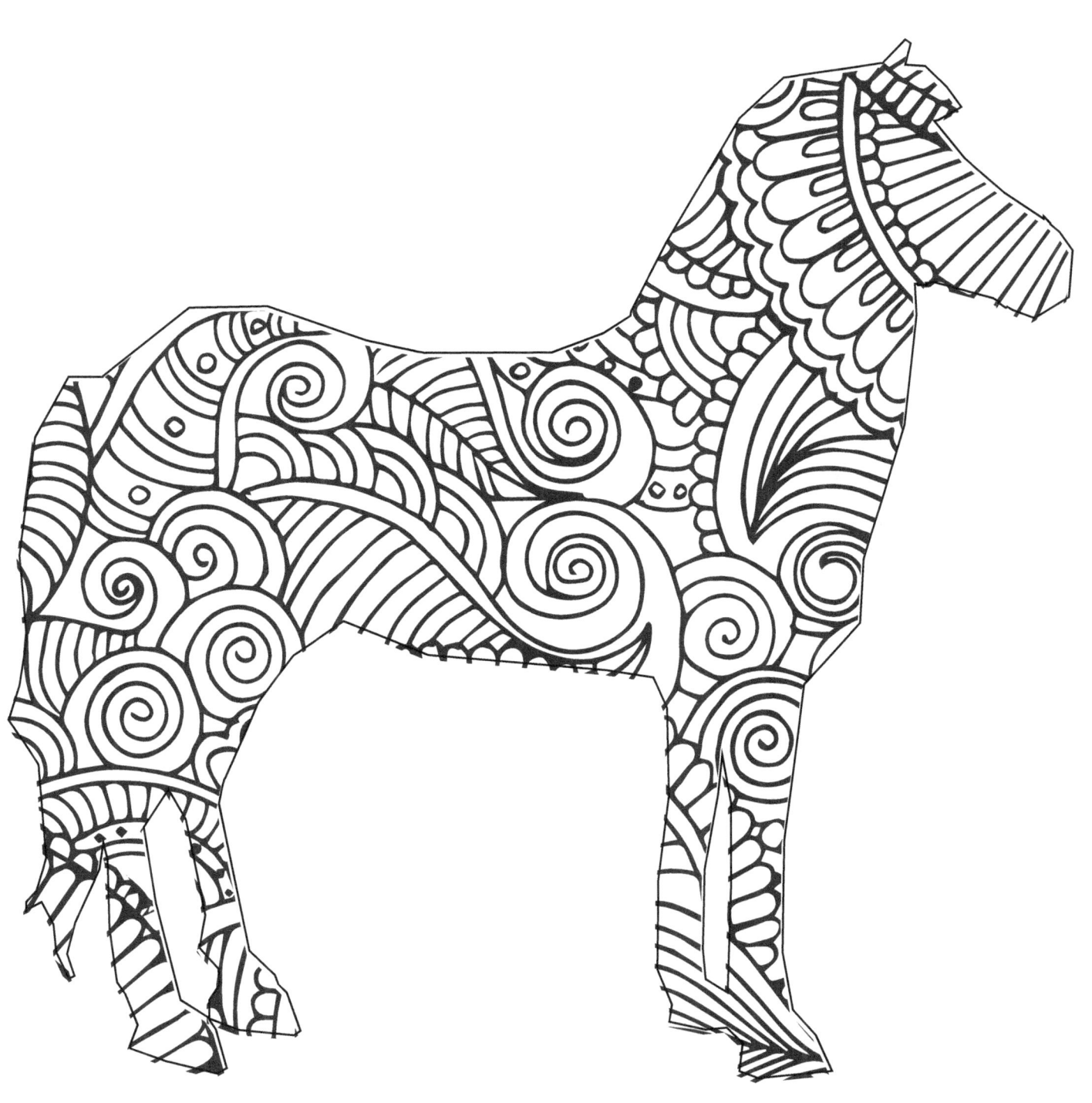

www.ingramcontent.com/pod-product-compliance
Lightning Source LLC
Chambersburg PA
CBHW080910220526
45466CB00011BA/3537